Thyroid POWER

Thyroid
POWER

Ten Steps
to Total Health

Richard L. Shames, M.D., *and*

Karilee H. Shames, R.N., Ph.D.

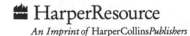

HarperResource

An Imprint of HarperCollins*Publishers*

FIRST EDITION

Designed by Jennifer Ann Daddio

Printed on acid-free paper

Library of Congress Cataloging-in-Publication Data
Shames, Richard.
Thyroid power : ten steps to total health / Richard L. Shames, and Karilee H. Shames.—1st ed.
p.   cm.
Includes bibliographical references and index.
ISBN 0-688-17236-9
1. Hypothyroidism—Popular works. I. Shames, Karilee Halo.
II. Title.

RC657 .S53 2001
616.4'44—dc21
00–053937

01   02   03   04   05   QW   10   9   8   7   6   5   4   3

Richard dedicates this book to Nathan Becker, M.D., endocrinology professor at UCSF Medical Center, for his many years of influential vision and clarity in advancing the importance of individualized thyroid care. Dr. Becker's refinements of Karilee's standard thyroid program led to such improvement in her quality of life that Richard was inspired to successfully incorporate these bold new ideas into his general practice.

Karilee dedicates this book to our three wonderful children: Shauna, Georjana, and Gabriel, for their laughter, wisdom, and loving support. May they continue to inspire all whose lives they touch.

Both authors dedicate this book to the millions who struggle with subtle low-thyroid conditions, in the hope that they find greater healing and wellness.

Contents

Acknowledgments

The authors gratefully acknowledge the following people for their invaluable contributions to this project:

Walter Maack, M.D., and David Chipkin, M.D., for their initial ideas regarding a needed book about thyroid, and Stuart Zoll, O.M.D., Centre for Preventive Medicine in Boca Raton, Florida, for his support during the final editing phase.

Michael Wanger, of Wanger Associates Video Productions in Kentfield, California, for his encouragement of the authors' multimedia efforts to share their technical information effectively.

Julia Ross, M.A., of Recovery Systems of Mill Valley, California, for her insistence that such a book would be valuable for the many people struggling with addictions, overweight, and eating disorders.

Associates from the American Holistic Nurses Association, especially Barbara Dossey, R.N., M.S., F.A.A.N., Lynn Keegan, R.N., Ph.D., F.A.A.N., plus Susan Luck, R.N., M.S., and Judy Lane, R.N., F.N.P., for their eternal friendship and support in our professional growth.

Karilee's colleagues at the Florida Atlantic University College of Nursing, particularly Eleanor Schuster, Ph.D., R.N., Debera Thomas Ph.D., R.N., and our Dean Anne Boykin, Ph.D., for their support in this educational project.

Faith Hamlin, our encouraging agent at Sanford Greenburger Associates, whose "faith" enabled this book to come to life.

Lana Thompson, of Vesalius Editing, in Boca Raton, Florida, who laboriously corrected and revised the manuscript.

Toni Sciarra, our careful and exacting senior editor at HarperCollins, whose patience and humor have guided our work.

In addition, we offer special gratitude to the women in Karilee's Thyroid Recovery Groups, for their long-term commitment to voicing and improving the many personal aspects of low thyroid conditions for themselves and for others.

Foreword

Hypothyroidism is undoubtedly the most common disorder of thyroid function. It affects both sexes and all ages; it may be overt or subclinical; the spectrum of severity is broad. At one extreme are patients who have a few symptoms and signs. At the other extreme are patients in coma. Hypothyroidism can be subclinical for many years, particularly in patients with autoimmune Hashimoto's thyroiditis.

Although we are beginning to understand immune mechanisms, we do not yet fully understand autoimmune thyroid disease. Hashimoto's disease is primarily cell-mediated immune destruction of the thyroid gland. In the less common Graves' disease (also called thyrotoxicosis), a circulating antibody drives the thyroid to hyperfunction, out of the control of pituitary TSH feedback. Graves' disease and Hashimoto's disease frequently coexist in families. Although the tendency to develop these autoimmune disorders is almost certainly inherited, we do not yet know *how* the malady is inherited.

What frequently confuses the average clinician is that patients often experience other autoimmune endocrinopathies simultaneously. Addison's disease (adrenal insufficiency), Type 1 diabetes (insulin dependent), autoimmune gonadal failure, hypoparathyroidism, and pituitary failure are not rare partners. Several years ago, Phyllis Saifer, M.D., and I coined the term APICH Syndrome, which introduced associative non-endocrine maladies with the previously outlined endocrine disorders. While clinically important, these relationships tantalized more than informed us about the basic mechanisms of autoimmunity.

Thyroid disorders are coupled maladies: localized inflammation with generalized flu-like symptoms, and resultant hormone excesses or deficiencies. It is no surprise that the patient, as well as the physician, is confused.

Amid this confusion, treatment with thyroid hormone—to the point of TSH suppression—is often diagnostic as well as therapeutic. These remarks would be considered heresy by academicians. Physicians and patients should, however, remember that academicians are often passionate, idealistic, eccentric, quarrelsome, and self-serving. They often do research, publish, teach, but rarely see or care for thyroid sufferers.

Regarding actual patient care, a trial of thyroid hormone therapy was often used to good advantage in the past. Today, with sensitive laboratory studies, such as TSH assays, our presumed ability to diagnose thyroid disease has encouraged the physician to treat the laboratory data instead of the patient. Consequently, empiric treatment with thyroid hormones has fallen out of favor.

Nevertheless, sensible, cost-effective treatments of widespread thyroid disorders remain an important concern of the physician, not least because the patient often presents with vague complaints that easily can be misdiagnosed. Patients who present with fatigue, depression, and subtle cognitive defects are frequently dismissed, discouraged, and mistreated. I've spent many years treating these patients with thyroxine (T-4) and more recently with concomitant triiodothyronine (T-3) with much success.

Regards and best wishes for your success as well,

—NATHAN BECKER, M.D., F.A.C.E., F.A.C.P.
Assistant Clinical Professor of Medicine
University of California at San Francisco

Low Thyroid: An Undeclared Epidemic

Although extremely common, low thyroid is largely an unsuspected illness. Even when suspected, it is frequently undiagnosed. When it is diagnosed, it often goes untreated. When it is treated, it is seldom treated optimally.

This book is intended to correct some of these shortcomings. Show this book to your health providers. Review some of the references. Ask questions and demand appropriate action. You deserve to feel strong, be healthy, and live fully.

How This Book Can Help

As a doctor-nurse team, we have spent more than twenty-five years helping people with the frustrating condition of borderline low thyroid. We became involved not only because so many of our patients were burdened with this life-sapping illness but also because Karilee and our three children have this genetic challenge.

This unusual book is the result of insight from a variety of sources, including other books, journals, conferences, and consultations with top university specialists. It is the first of its kind to provide an actual step-by-step program that allows you to tackle this complex and deceptive syndrome one layer at a time. Consider it a long, personal visit with a caring, prevention-oriented practitioner. Let it guide you on a journey from a set of diverse symptoms, seemingly unconnected, to a definite diagnosis and effective treatment.

Ten simple steps will show you how to create a more effective healing program and become an empowered health care consumer. In addition to improving low thyroid, our overall approach to healing might be useful with other conditions.

Each of the ten steps can be a journey in itself. For those who wish to "jump right in," we have included a 5-Day Jump Start. For those who wish to pursue complementary methods of healing, there is a special section called "Beyond the Tenth Step." For those who wish to collaborate with their physician on this journey, we have included a research-based section called "Show This to Your Doctor," which provides scientific documentation to support each step.

For us, a whole-person approach to low thyroid is one of the most exciting areas in all of medicine. It is our intent to prompt additional research into this vitally important topic.

The journey to reclaim your full vitality can be one of life's most fulfilling experiences. If you suffer from low thyroid, it is our deepest wish that you enjoy a healthier and more satisfying existence, one that allows you to make your greatest contribution to the world.

You now have in your possession a helpful road map. You are in the driver's seat, and we are delighted to travel this road with you. Enjoy the ride!

Consider Thyroid the Hidden Factor in Your Overall Health

The energy to live a full adult living breathing life in close contact with what I love—I want to enter into it, and be part of it.
—KATHERINE MANSFIELD, in her journal, 1922

Karilee's Story

I led a normal life until the birth of my second daughter. I was thirty-two, professionally accomplished, and enjoying myself except for one problem—I was so tired, I could hardly get out of bed. I felt constantly exhausted. I blamed it on having young children and perhaps a touch of postpartum depression. The doctors I saw tried to convince me that this was normal, although I couldn't understand how other mothers could live like that. I had no energy for life and felt depleted and irritable. I had no interest in recreation or sex, which eventually began to affect our marital relationship. I was too tired even to care!

I was also experiencing some strange symptoms that no one could explain. In addition to weight gain, I had exceptionally dry skin and hair and brittle nails. I also began to suffer from migraine headaches, which incapacitated me for twenty-four to forty-eight hours, once a month, and left me feeling completely drained. Another most unsettling symptom, which plagued me for many months, was a thick tongue that I would bite many times a day, without knowing why or what to do about it.

I had no idea that I was another unsuspecting victim of an increasingly common medical ailment. Neither did my doctors. Like many new mothers, I simply felt tired. My energy was low, accompanied by some annoying symptoms. My checkups and regular tests were normal. I did not have anemia, AIDS, mononucleosis, or depression. What I did have, however, was a growing inability to fully enjoy life.

Fortunately, one practitioner caring for me had the wisdom to consider the possibility of thyroid problems and did some testing. My levels of thyroid hormone were low. We began to experiment with Synthroid, a synthetic thyroid pill, and after several months of trying different doses, hit upon one that made a definite difference. I began to feel human again.

For me, it has been a long, slow journey. There have been times, perhaps even years, when I could forget about this metabolic challenge. At other times, most notably when there has been additional physical or emotional stress in my life, I have found myself highly symptomatic. That inconsistency makes responding to this challenge an even more delicate process, requiring professional monitoring. When I am plagued with some of the symptoms, such as irritability or depression, it is often my close associates who remind me to explore my metabolism. I tend to think "it's just me. I'm having a tough day/week/month." It is easy to forget that I have a delicate hormonal dance going on inside, one that requires continual rebalancing.

Rest assured that my situation is exceedingly common. In the last twenty-five years of our practicing general medicine/nursing, one of the most common illnesses we treat is a type of low energy. We are not speaking about simple fatigue from lack of sleep or overwork. We are talking about a profound low energy, one that does not seem to improve easily with rest. It is beyond simple exhaustion; it is a medical situation.

Alma's Story

Let's consider another example. Even climbing the short flight of stairs to our office seemed overwhelming to Alma. Her face spoke of exhaustion. In the examining room, she presented her complaints: "Fatigue; decreased concentration; weight gain; depression; anxiety; vague migrating aches and pains; feeling too hot some of the time, and at other times too cold." Alma had already been examined by more than one internist, who all agreed that she needed to be seen by a psychiatrist. All these visits had been costly, time consuming, and unhelpful. None had addressed the underlying cause.

Alma's depression and anxiety were not so much mental problems as they were the result of a medical problem, one that is repeatedly undiagnosed. To us it was an open-and-shut case of low thyroid.

Alma is only one of the thousands of people we've seen in recent years whose blood tests are normal and who wonder if they are going crazy. They have traveled from doctor to doctor, pharmacy to pharmacy, sometimes even trying a variety of alternative treatments, all to no avail. According to a recent survey by the University of Colorado, "Investigators have found the prevalence of mild thyroid failure to be approximately 10% in the general population and up to 20% in older women."[1]

Doctors on the thyroid service at the Harvard Medical School agree that the incidence of the disorder is one woman out of every twelve under age fifty. By age sixty it is one woman out of every six.[2] It is common knowledge that one-fifth of the U.S. population is overweight, and countless others suffer from a variety of eating disorders that could well be connected to thyroid problems. Millions of people are depressed and many are taking antidepressant medication. (For many years, Prozac has been the number one best selling prescription drug.) Millions of adults suffer from low energy, while we are faced with an epidemic of attention deficit disorder and hyperactive children. Little attention has been given to the mechanism of these maladies. We believe—and many other researchers concur—that much of it can be related to abnormal thyroid function.

Other experts estimate that at any given time, more than half of those with low-grade hypothyroidism remain undiagnosed. This means that an enormous number of people might have a story similar to Karilee's or Alma's. In 1999, Synthroid, the medicine most commonly prescribed for low thyroid, became the number one bestselling prescription drug. Thus, we are clearly dealing with a large-scale epidemic that has been inadequately addressed.

Lessons from Other Epidemics

In ancient Rome, doctors were baffled by an illness that appeared gradually and then grew into an epidemic. Apparently, increasing numbers of people began to act in bizarre ways. (An example is the behavior of Emperor Nero, who allegedly fiddled while Rome burned.) The illness presented as mild gastrointestinal symptoms accompanied by an unusual form of dementia. Ancient Roman doctors were astute about human illness, yet despite their judicious application of medical information, they were mystified about the cause.

The mystery was solved only in recent years, through bone mineral studies performed on human remains found in the catacombs beneath Rome. Some of these bones, dated to the era of the mysterious malady, were found to contain an inordinately high level of lead. Evidently, the epidemic had been lead poisoning, the symptoms of which are indeed dementia and gastrointestinal distress.

How did lead poisoning become so widespread? Those beautiful Roman aqueducts, some of which still stand in southern Europe, were lined with lead piping. The water, as it traveled, picked up lead contamination. In addition, many people used lead utensils for cooking and eating, leading to contamination of their food. Historians estimate that the Roman empire at its height refined nearly a hundred thousand tons of lead every year.

The upper classes of society suffered the most from this epidemic. They could afford the fancier lead utensils and mountain water delivered by the aqueducts. The lower classes used mostly pottery and obtained their water from local streams. They seemed to experience this illness less. Some intelligent people in Rome noticed this class distinction. They adopted some of the customs of the lower class as a way of avoiding this mysterious illness.

Another epidemic, called the plague, occurred in the Middle Ages. It was caused by bacterial infection spread mostly by fleas, but often by coughing or sneezing. Once again, medical authorities of the time could not determine the true cause of the terrible disease.

There was, however, one minor religious order whose participants believed that the plague was caused by little devils too small to be seen. These people advocated wearing a mask, stuffed with cotton, in front of the nose and mouth, intended to keep the tiny devils out. As you might imagine, this maneuver worked quite well against airborne plague. Long before the scientific discovery of bacteria, some people managed to remain free from the epidemic.

These stories have a moral. It may take years before we understand all the reasons for our present thyroid epidemic, but we can start doing smart things right now to handle its debilitating symptoms. Let us begin with a better understanding of the basic illness itself.

What Exactly Is Low Thyroid Disease?

Our country is in the grip of yet another energy crisis. Both men and women are working harder, demanding more of themselves, and are pressured to get more done in less time. With the increased pace of life and the increased chemical contamination of our air, food, and water, people are more than simply work-exhausted or stressed out. Many are actually developing a chronic, low-energy illness.

One of the most common places for this energy illness to strike is the thyroid gland, a butterfly-shaped, hormone-producing tissue at the lower front of the neck. It is walnut-size, located just below the Adam's apple. When this gland is hampered by illness, causing reduced production of thyroid hormone, every bodily function is diminished. This is because every cell in the body needs small amounts of thyroid hormone to function optimally.

People vary in just what functions are diminished most when thyroid hormone is low. For some, the function most affected is energy level. For others, it is body temperature. For still others, it can be personality (low mood) or lowered resistance to infection. Some people have many symptoms, while others have only a few. Regardless of the number of symptoms, the lay term for the condition is low thyroid.

The medical terminology, however, is more complex, and diagnosis depends on ascertaining just *why* the gland is underproducing thyroid hormone. This is the crux of the whole issue. Why would one of the body's most important endocrine glands start slowing its production at a time when full operation is needed more than ever? Let's take a closer look.

The thyroid gland can be viewed as a tiny but powerful throttle mechanism, because the energy hormone it produces acts like a gas pedal for the rest of the body. The hormone circulates through the bloodstream and enters each cell. Then, in the presence of thyroid hormone, a complex protein molecule binds to DNA in a different manner than it would without the presence of thyroid hormone. This entire mechanism described above functions like a toggle switch to turn cellular machinery on or off. In doing this, it regulates cell temperature, cell function, and cell growth.

The thyroid gland, therefore, controls every chemical reaction of every organ in the body. Without it, the body would cool off and slow down to the point of death. One can get along without a uterus or a prostate gland, or without ovaries, testes, or even a kidney. One cannot survive without thyroid hormone. A person whose thyroid gland is removed needs a daily supplement of thyroid hormone.

Low thyroid conditions do not cause people to die. Instead they cause people to feel half-dead, or sometimes to wish they were dead. The symptoms range from annoying to debilitating, with many people experiencing a severity somewhere in between. As we have said, the illness is frustrating, surprisingly common, and alarmingly on the increase. In fact, this condition could rapidly become known as the disease of our time.

The little thyroid gland manages to do a big job by combining two rather simple substances, which together make thyroid hormone. One of these is iodine. This common element is naturally abundant in foods from the oceans and coastal regions of the planet, but is more scarce inland.

Worldwide, the cause of most low thyroid function is low dietary iodine. In other words, low thyroid occurs when a person is not consuming enough iodine to make sufficient quantities of thyroid hormone to fuel the body cells. In our country, however, low iodine has ceased to be the cause of low thyroid function, because extra iodine is put into various foodstuffs, including table salt and bread dough.

The second substance needed to make thyroid hormone is tyrosine, a common amino acid found in most proteins. Amino acids are simple organic molecules, either manufactured easily in the body or obtained from the digestion of protein in the diet. Tyrosine is so abundant that a lack of it cannot be causing the widespread low thyroid epidemic seen in industrialized nations.

No, our present epidemic of low thyroid is not due to a shortage of the raw material, or building blocks, needed to make thyroid hormone. Instead, there seems to be some disruption in the assembly phase. Normally, these building blocks undergo a series of reactions in the thyroid gland, resulting in the attachment of four atoms of iodine to one molecule of tyrosine. This product is called T-4 or thyroxine. A more complete name for T-4 is levo-thyroxine, or simply l-thyroxine. It is one of the two main thyroid hormones and the one most commonly measured. T-4 is carried around in the circulation bound to special blood proteins. It is considered the slow-acting or "storage" thyroid hormone, because in its circulating form it cannot bind to the cell nucleus material.

It is instead T-3 that acts as the gas pedal for the DNA cell machinery. T-4 gives up one atom of iodine to make T-3, fast-acting or "active" thyroid hormone. Its full name is triiodothyronine, or simply thyronine. Even though its role in the body seems supreme, it is currently measured less often and is less often used in thyroid pills than the better-known T-4.

The production of thyroid hormone in the body is elegantly controlled by brain signals to the pituitary gland. This tiny gland at the base of the brain regulates the thyroid gland in the neck by means of the chemical TSH or thyroid stimulating hormone, a pituitary chemical whose level in the blood reveals the brain's satisfaction with thyroid production.

Low thyroid symptoms occur when the body tissues do not get enough of either T-4 or T-3 or both, apparently because of disrupted assembly within the thyroid gland. Generations of scientists have studied this disruption, but only recently have they discovered the actual mechanism for the problem.

It turns out that the cause of virtually all cases of low thyroid is not so much a faulty thyroid gland as it is an overzealous immune system. As strange as it may seem, common low thyroid is a mild immune system illness in which the immune system wrongly attacks the innocent thyroid gland. The illness is called Hashimoto's thyroiditis in honor of the Japanese doctor who first identified it.

Of course, there are other kinds of thyroid problems: infections, injuries, benign nodules, and cancer, for instance. But most simple low thyroid disease is immune caused.[3] In later steps, we'll discuss some of these other thyroid conditions, but our main focus will be on the most prevalent challenge by far: simple low thyroid.

How Is the Immune System Involved?

Normally, the immune system is poised and waiting to defend the body against foreign invaders such as viruses or bacteria. Part of this job involves constant search-and-destroy missions by certain white blood cells called neutrophils and monocytes. These cells are always in motion, hunting down a hiding germ or cleaning up cellular debris. On a good day, they can even direct a killer lymphocyte into eliminating a previously normal body cell that has recently turned cancerous.

All this normal immune function is, of course, to our benefit. We live in a veritable sea of bacteria and other creepy-crawlies that are nicely held at bay by the relentless and vigilant immune system. However, some of us pay a price for its pervasive vigilance. Without warning and for no good reason, our immune system can sometimes start attacking our normal cells and tissues.

It is clearly a mistake for the body to attack itself, but it does happen. The name for this seemingly bizarre event is autoimmune illness. Once thought to be rare, it is now known to be surprisingly common. No longer is the list of autoimmune illnesses limited to rare conditions such as lupus, myasthenia, sarcoidosis, or scleroderma. Now it has been determined that very common diseases such as diabetes, rheumatoid arthritis, and possibly Parkinson's disease are autoimmune in nature. In fact, very recent data suggests that multiple sclerosis is also an autoimmune illness. For all we know, even Alzheimer's, now this country's fourth leading cause of death among the elderly, could eventually be identified as an autoimmune illness. Added to all this is the enormous incidence of autoimmune thyroid. The fact is, autoimmune problems have reached epidemic proportions.

How did so many immune systems get so unbalanced? Step 9 of this book is fully devoted to this question. For the moment, let us say that recent research is suggesting runaway environmental pollutants, among others, as likely culprits. These deleterious influences appear to be assaulting our sensitive and delicately balanced immune systems, causing mixed messages within the body. Some of the new chemicals our immune system tries to fend off are hormone mimics. Others are hormone blockers. Still others are immune disrupters. Many of the thousands of these new chemicals dumped into the environment are simply low-level poisons.

In a desperate attempt to ward off an apparent assault from all sides, our confused antibodies are increasingly attacking our own glands and hormones. No one knows the exact mechanism, but the results are becoming obvious. The most common result is a mild or moderately inflamed thyroid gland, producing suboptimal amounts of active hormone. The long list of physical and mental symptoms arising from a lowered thyroid hormone level is summarized at the end of this step and is expanded in Step 3.

Why Is Autoimmune Thyroid Disease Becoming More Common?

There is compelling evidence that today's thyroid epidemic is multi-factored, rather than due to chemical agents alone. In other words, various nonchemical factors might be combining with the chemical siege to cause our immune systems to make antibodies against our own thyroid glands. If you have a family history of low thyroid, diabetes, or other rheumatic/autoimmune illness, then almost any serious physical or mental stress might trigger the primed immune system into mischievous action against the thyroid, one of its favorite body targets.

Other than genetics and chemicals, are there other risk factors that could account for the low-energy epidemic? Could radiation, for example, be another cause? We know how deleterious this can be on sensitive immune balance. With the depletion of the ozone layer, our exposure to the sun's ultraviolet radiation is increasing. What about our exposure to whatever radiation is emitted by cell phones, computer screens, or countertop microwave ovens? Do you suppose this exposure is on the increase?

Not only is the neck a likely place to receive much of this added new radiation, but the thyroid gland is particularly sensitive to it. Even more directly sensitizing to the delicate thyroid is the increased irrigation of food crops with brackish water containing significant amounts of radioactive iodine 131. This potentially toxic isotope is known to head straight for the thyroid gland and become concentrated there.

One nonchemical immune irritant that may be on the increase is intestinal parasites. Once thought to be a problem confined to third world populations, a wide variety of mild parasitic conditions now affects the average city dweller in the United States. Sometimes, without causing severe distress, their presence is like a thorn in the side of the immune system, which makes increased levels of antibodies against them. Increased antibody production against the parasites has a subtle way of spilling over into increased antibody production against the thyroid.

Still another possibly suspicious trend on the increase is the widespread fluoridation of municipal water supplies. This well-intended activity has been so widely accepted in today's society that it is shocking to read the mounting research casting doubt on its safety. The short-range goal of reducing tooth decay seems to have blinded many to the long-range risks to sensitive immune balance posed by fluoridation. We'll discuss these and other risks in detail in Steps 8 and 9.

The high stress of daily life may be as big a factor in thyroid disease as it is in heart disease. Anxiety and depression are known to have deleterious effects on immune balance. Also, the increasingly rapid pace of life may leave little time for immune-restoring activities such as aerobic exercise, muscle building, or slow stretching. What is disruptive to the immune system now may be disruptive to a thyroid gland later.

According to medical textbooks, these complex and subtle issues are medically significant. They may all be contributing to the higher prevalence of this enormous autoimmune problem.

Richard saw one of these effects firsthand. A few years ago, he was asked to serve on an ad hoc medical committee in the San Francisco area. A major oil company had accidentally released an unusual chemical mix into the air above its refinery. The nearby isolated town of Crockett, population 3,000, was soon covered with a misty shower of a supposedly nonpoisonous substance known as catacarb.

Within hours, people were flooding local emergency rooms seeking relief from disturbing skin, eye, and nasal symptoms. These initial symptoms resolved over a period of days or weeks with treatment and a healthier lifestyle, although the heightened allergic responses lasted for several months longer.

One major health effect, however, does not seem to be resolving but is intensifying especially in people who made no lifestyle modifications. A large segment of the population exposed to the chemical spill is experiencing a gradual reduction in thyroid function. This reduction is almost certain to be autoimmune glandular disease, triggered by acute chemical exposure. Although the acute toxicity was soon gone, it must have triggered the delicate workings of the immune system into an ongoing response.

Similar but milder events could be taking place in other locations around the country, as the result of various other kinds of exposure. Thus, we all may need to learn some simple, effective ways to respond to these episodic chemical onslaughts against our immune/glandular system, for surely there will be more toxic assaults in the future.

How Does Low Thyroid Masquerade as Other Illness?

Certain other autoimmune illnesses are often easier to diagnose than low thyroid. They occur in isolated parts of the body, such as in knee inflammation. The joint swells, then becomes hot, red, and tender. Simple blood tests such as the sedimentation rate and the rheumatoid factor show up as abnormal. The person suffering these symptoms is given a diagnosis of rheumatoid arthritis and treatment is started.

However, suppose your autoimmune response involves an attack on your thyroid gland. The gland itself and blood tests may not show any abnormalities. You may instead exhibit a complex array of bizarre symptoms, which don't fit any common pattern. Your major symptom might be physical exhaustion. Or, it could be anxiety or lack of concentration. Even insomnia, often attributed to excess worrying, can be low thyroid's sole presenting complaint.

In the scenario above, instead of an accurate diagnosis and effective treatment, we have an ongoing nagging problem. The initial symptom of fatigue may progress and affect specific body systems. For example, an increasingly sluggish intestine may cause a high degree of indigestion, gas, or constipation. Your doctor may prescribe treatments for these symptoms. The now sluggish liver may cause abnormally high cholesterol and triglyceride levels, resulting in still other treatments. Sluggish skin can erupt in acne or eczema, or suffer with severe dryness or a host of typical or atypical rashes. Once again, doctors have many diagnoses and treatments for these symptoms. The same scenario is played out with headaches, recurring infections, minor eye complaints, heart palpitations, and balance problems.

Perhaps the biggest potential for mischief is in the arena of women's health. Everything from minor vaginal irritations to repeated miscarriages has been shown to be thyroid-related in a certain percentage of sufferers. Endometriosis is frequently a key indicator of a low thyroid problem.

Many women in our practice are experiencing what seems like another epidemic: infertility. Many of these clients have spent thousands of hours—and dollars—in desperate attempts to become pregnant. When nothing else has worked, a large percentage have responded beautifully and quickly to the simple addition of thyroid hormone. In these cases, autoimmune low thyroid was the real cause of the infertility. How many other illnesses are being treated suboptimally because low thyroid is being missed?

Menopause is not an illness, but it can surely begin to feel that way if your thyroid is low or borderline at the time of your change. In such a situation, which is extremely common, the insomnia, hot flashes, mood swings, and night sweats can be debilitatingly severe. Generally, low progesterone is an underlying issue as well.

Women in this frustrating circumstance are often told, "It's just your low estrogen from menopause," as if they should expect to feel awful for years because of a natural reduction in estrogen. Without an accurate diagnosis of low thyroid, or low progesterone, these women are simply given estrogen, a thyroid inhibiter, and their symptoms linger. The ovaries and uterus need proper amounts of thyroid hormone as much as the skin and liver do. Step 6 will discuss the effects of thyroid hormones on women's health.

Low thyroid masquerading as mental illness is quite possibly an even bigger issue. Frequently, and unfortunately for many, a low level of thyroid hormone may yield no physical signs or symptoms whatever. Instead what you get is low thyroid causing low brain function.

One of the most common symptoms is depression. Some studies have shown that over half the people treated by doctors for depression have low thyroid as a cause of their condition. Thus, many who are currently taking Prozac and other powerful antidepressants might do better by taking thyroid medication in place of or in conjunction with their mood medication.

Anxiety, panic attacks, attention deficit disorder, phobias, dementia, increased sleepiness, loss of ambition, and several other moods have been linked to abnormalities in thyroid gland or thyroid hormone function. Even relationship stress can trigger a thyroid imbalance, and vice versa. All too frequently, the underlying problem is missed.

Why Is Thyroid Diagnosis So Often Missed?

The answer is simple. First, the standard lab tests are unable to identify the millions of borderline low thyroid sufferers. Inadequate testing results in inaccurate diagnosis. Thyroid tests are designed to show a positive result for a thyroid abnormality. They will not show a positive result for any other illness, so an abnormal result can be trusted. The problem, however, is with the normal results. The thyroid tests used today are just not sensitive enough to identify mild thyroid failure. You could be uncomfortably low in thyroid and still show normal in tests. Individuals differ in what is "normal" for them.

Over and over, people come to us from other doctors with no clear diagnosis for their low energy or other symptoms. When they got their checkup, they were told that everything was fine and that even their blood tests were within normal range. They were then told, "Oh, it's just you. You're a low-energy person," or even that they were simply depressed or menopausal.

So they kept on trudging along, dragging through each day. They drank more coffee, ate more sweets, and hoped that things would get better, or at least not get too much worse. Their actual medical condition went undiagnosed for many years. Because of current testing trends, they would have to become really sick with low thyroid before it could be diagnosed.

It is possible, however, that the problem is not with the testing technology, but with the test interpretation. When blood tests are read, the range defined as normal for thyroid is so wide that it includes almost everyone, disregarding the unique metabolic needs of each person. Those diagnosed as really sick are actually only the tip of a large iceberg. There are many, many more who are mildly to moderately affected. These people can feel miserable for years with a variety of minor complaints that can keep a group of specialists quite busy, each surveying and treating the problem from their own limited perspective. The sufferers are therefore frequently shuffled from specialist to specialist, paying enormous bills, gradually feeling worse, and perhaps eventually becoming despondent.

Now, with the added constraints of managed care, doctors are spending less and less time with each patient, and are therefore even less likely to accurately diagnose a mild or subtle medical situation. In the past, the patient might have been referred to an endocrinologist, who would take the extra time to figure out the problem. Today, however, only acutely ill people are referred to a specialist, leaving a high percentage who are not in imminent danger of dying but are suffering ongoing marginal health.

In a medical system geared to catastrophic illness and crisis intervention, the common milder cases of low thyroid generally go undiagnosed. Sadly, most people probably do not even realize that low energy could be a treatable medical problem. The major symptoms of thyroid disease are so common today as to be considered normal: low energy, marginal health, and overweight.

Generally, people figure their sluggishness is simply a result of excess stress, inactivity, or lack of sleep. While that might be partly true, more often people have trouble sleeping, exercising, or managing stress because of this metabolic malfunction.

This brings up another reason why proper diagnosis is often missed. Patients are not generally aware that these common symptoms could be medically significant. Therefore they do not even think to bring them up to their doctor.

Sometimes, on the other hand, a patient with a long list of mild symptoms is dismissed by the doctor as a hypochondriac. Women especially tend to receive this kind of label, even being called "hysterical."

How This Book Can Help: The Step-by-Step Plan for Total Thyroid Health

This book presents a step-by-step approach to healing low thyroid. Early steps reveal the scope of the problem and who is most likely to suffer from low thyroid. The middle steps explain what we believe are the best standard and not-so-standard treatments that modern medicine can offer. Next, we discuss how the ovaries and adrenal glands are affected by low thyroid, and which tests and medicines are needed to treat these problems. Then we detail which alternative treatments are most helpful and exactly what you can do for optimal management of an autoimmune disease. Finally, in Step 10, we review the best health ideas we know for living a thyroid-friendly lifestyle. Then we present a plan for using these ten steps to actualize your highest potential.

If you, or someone you care about, is in what we call a thyroid dilemma, this book can help immensely. We think that our holistic approach fills an important gap by viewing illness from a multidimensional perspective, including nutrition, exercise, stress reduction, and spiritual awareness. You may need to decrease your exposure to toxic chemicals. You may need to decrease your exposure to toxic people. You may even need to decrease your exposure to toxic health providers! Our step-by-step approach will help start you on the path to health and well-being. We wish you good traveling on your journey.

Low thyroid is only one type of low energy. Karilee and Alma have this type. You may have a different or additional diagnosis. You will need to explore and consider various other types of energy depletion. Some simple and easy ways to accomplish this are presented in Step 2.

Do You Have Low Thyroid? A Self-Assessment

The following questionnaire provides an initial opportunity for you to determine if your situation is suspicious for low thyroid. Step 3 offers a more detailed evaluation to help you and your practitioner determine if low thyroid is your likely diagnosis.

If you have already been diagnosed and/or treated for low thyroid you should still take this little quiz. A troubling percentage of treated patients continue to have thyroid-related symptoms, even after their blood tests return to normal. They clearly need some of the additional treatments outlined in this book.

Do you . . .

____ have unusual fatigue unrelated to exertion?

____ feel chillier than most people, often needing to wear socks to bed?

____ dress in layers because of needing to adjust to various temperatures throughout the day (sometimes too hot, sometimes too cold)?

____ have feelings of anxiety that sometimes lead to panic?

____ have trouble with weight, often eating lightly, yet still not losing a pound?

____ experience aches and pains in your muscles and joints unrelated to trauma or exercise?

____ have increased problems with digestion or allergies?

____ feel mentally sluggish, unfocused, or unusually forgetful, even though you're not old enough to have Alzheimer's?

____ know of anyone in your family who has ever had a thyroid problem (even yourself at an earlier age)?

____ suffer from dry skin, or are prone to adult acne or eczema?

____ go through periods of depression, and/or lowered sex drive, seemingly out of proportion to life events?

____ have diabetes, anemia, rheumatoid arthritis, or early graying of hair? Does anyone in your family?

____ experience your hair as feeling like straw, dry and easily falling out?

____ experience significant menopausal symptoms, including migraine headaches, without full relief after taking estrogen?

____ have a history of whiplash or other neck injuries (which may have damaged your thyroid)?

____ have significant exposure, now or in the past, to chlorine, bromine, or fluoride (which compete with iodine in your thyroid)?

____ feel utterly exhausted by evening, yet have trouble sleeping? ✓

____ Do you wake up tired? ✓

If you answered yes to four or more of these questions, you could be one of millions of people with an undiagnosed or under-treated low thyroid problem. Keep reading, and be sure to take the self-assessment in Step 3, as well as the recommended blood and temperature tests, to help determine if low thyroid is your definite diagnosis. Once your situation is diagnosed, it can then be treated optimally, using some of the suggestions in this book. Good luck!

Learn How Low Thyroid Makes Any Illness Worse

We have now crossed a threshold to the point where we can effectively diagnose and treat your fatigue.
—JACOB TEITELBAUM, M.D, *From Fatigued to Fantastic*

Could symptoms that seem like low thyroid actually be a result of another low-energy disease? Of course. Could these same symptoms actually be from a combination of low thyroid *and* some other energy-sapping disease? Certainly. There are many additional causes of fatigue and marginal health, each requiring a different treatment.

Coexistent low thyroid can worsen any other illness, and—interestingly enough—the opposite is also true. To achieve lasting improvement, you may have to treat more than one condition at a time. It is critical that you obtain a full and complete diagnosis and treat in the appropriate order all conditions that may be contributing to your health dilemma. While simple low energy is often a common condition with an easy resolution, it can sometimes be maddeningly deceptive and hard to diagnose.

The first, critical step is to find a qualified health care practitioner with whom to collaborate. You have a right, as a health consumer, to fully understand your condition, to hear the range of possible treatments, and to assess their benefits and detriments prior to making any decisions. Ultimately, it is you who must direct your journey toward health. Achieving a proper diagnosis is a critical beginning step that can save years of pain and anguish.

Finding a Doctor Who Understands

As health professionals, we are extremely supportive of personal empowerment and self-care. However, in addition to books, friends, and the Internet, it is essential to secure the help of a trained professional. A good practitioner can properly assist you in diagnosing the true cause of marginal health or significant low energy, saving you years of distress, unnecessary treatments, expense, and hardship.

A knowledgeable practitioner takes a complete history, listening carefully to nuances and identifying patterns. Then, he or she performs the proper physical examination and orders appropriate laboratory tests to ascertain exactly what kind of low energy you have so as to accurately determine which treatments will be most helpful. Don't sell yourself short. Make sure from the beginning to have your condition properly diagnosed.

Since low energy is a very common problem, many doctors hear this complaint often and have a standard, preset way of approaching it. Generally, if the fatigue does not seem severe to the practitioner, he or she will simply offer some reassurance. This can take the form of a little pep talk that acknowledges the financial squeeze people may be feeling, the hectic pace of modern life, and the difficulty in getting enough exercise, proper diet, and rest.

If you want to get beyond the simple pep talk, you will need to be very clear about how to present your symptoms to your physician. Write down everything that bothers you and the degree to which it interferes with your life. List the associated difficulties, if any, and describe as objectively as possible how the productivity in your life is being affected. If you feel noticeably less productive at work than you did a couple of years ago, make a note of this, and be specific.

If you have trouble getting started in the morning and arrive late at the office, mention that. If it used to take one cup of coffee to get started, and it now takes three, indicate this. If you can only get to your job site with great difficulty, dragging yourself out of bed and through the morning routine, definitely mention it. Explain what an imposition this is on the quality and enjoyment of your life. If you run out of steam at three or four P.M. but still have to work several more hours, describe briefly how hard this is for you, and what a sense of limitation you are feeling. If you can make it through the day but have no energy for evening activities, even enjoyable ones such as dinner and a movie, then mention how this "disability" is causing you some real distress and concern.

If other people are suffering in some way because of your fatigue, such as a spouse, children, or elderly loved ones who need more care and attention than you can provide, mention that clearly and objectively. Describe the emotions this lack of energy may be causing in terms of anger, frustration, or even despair. Make it apparent how much aggravation and irritation low energy is causing in your life. Try to quantify how your daily life is different from a few months or years ago. Try to pinpoint when and how your health began to change. Keep records that can portray the problem, even creating visual graphs if necessary to demonstrate changes in your health and ability to perform or enjoy your life.

It is imperative that, as a health consumer, you direct the course of the appointment with your health provider. The more assertive, clear, and focused you can be, the more likely you are to have your needs met in a timely and satisfactory fashion. Most people find it advantageous to write down questions prior to their appointment, even prioritizing their concerns so that if they run out of time, the major considerations will have been addressed. If you do not understand something you are being told or asked to do, don't be embarrassed to ask questions and get your needs met. Remember, you are your own best health advocate in these situations.

If you have obtained information from friends or websites related to your condition, it would be a good idea to share this with your practitioner to obtain further input. In these instances, be alert to the response of your practitioner. If your doctor acts as if your questions are a bother or doesn't answer directly, consider whether you are receiving optimal treatment. If your doctor doesn't know the answers, ask if he or she can find out for you, or direct you to the proper resource. You may need to shop for the right practitioner, just as you would shop for the right mechanic, contractor, or other service you value.

Seeing the Whole Picture: Low-Energy Conditions That May Be Thyroid-Related

We mentioned that you could have other conditions that compound or are compounded by low thyroid. Two conditions, in particular—

low ovary and low adrenal—will each be discussed in a step of their own later in this book. We discuss others below.

Anemic Without Knowing It

If you have too little iron in your diet, you may have the medical condition called iron deficiency anemia. (Iron is a key building block of the oxygen-carrying protein in red blood cells called hemoglobin). You could be feeling extremely sluggish, having many of the symptoms of low thyroid. In reality, you may simply need to take some iron supplements, or ingest iron-rich foods, to boost your red blood cell count back to normal.

As with any significant step in your health care journey, make sure to consult a health care practitioner before taking iron supplements. Iron is one of the few nutrients which, when ingested in excessive amounts, can lead to harmful overdose, especially in men.

There are other causes of anemia besides low iron. Sometimes anemia sufferers are lacking vitamin B_{12}, or another B vitamin called folic acid. A deficiency of these vitamins is as easy to correct as an iron deficiency. In addition to fatigue, symptoms of anemia include chilliness, pallor, and weakness. The physical examination for anemia is rather straightforward at the doctor's office, but you could be mildly anemic and have nothing show up on the physical examination.

The blood test for anemia is the simplest and least expensive of all blood tests, as well as one of the most accurate. The test which measures white cells too is called a complete blood count (CBC). Sometimes, in addition, the doctor will order a test for the blood iron level. A recent improvement in that determination is called a ferretin level. If anemia is found, the simple corrective measures we've already mentioned are often helpful, although sometimes the evaluation and treatment can be more complex. For example, sometimes a person with anemia has low thyroid. In this case, the low thyroid can be partially, or totally, causing the anemia, due to sluggish production of red blood cells and sluggish absorption of iron from the intestine.

Low Energy Due to Low Thyroid Versus Fatigue from Lack of Sleep
One simple reason for low energy is lack of sleep. People are working longer, driving themselves harder, and as a result are sleeping less than the seven to nine hours that many need. Many people also don't sleep as well at night because of anxiety from the day's stresses. In addition, some of the products we use to reduce stress can actually interfere with sleep patterns. These include caffeine, alcohol, tobacco, and sugar.

Fatigue due to lack of sleep is not easy to pinpoint in physical exams or in blood tests, and many doctors fail to question their patients carefully. One interesting strategy would be to start getting one hour more of sleep per night and see how you're feeling at the end of one week. If you're feeling substantially better, part of your fatigue—perhaps a large part of it—might be due to lack of sufficient sleep.

General Malnutrition Despite Eating Too Much
If, however, after getting more sleep, you still feel like you're dragging through three feet of water most of the day, your fatigue may be due to something else. General malnutrition, which goes beyond the simple iron deficiency that causes low energy, might be a culprit. It can be characterized by a deficiency of any one of a great many other minerals, vitamins, or amino acids.

With people working as hard as they do, there is less time to shop for and prepare nutritious food. Some people have become so accustomed to relying on fast food that they eat it almost exclusively—french fries from the drive-up window, pizza ordered in, or waffles from the freezer. Whatever the case, the result is the same—you could be malnourished even though you eat a lot of food and may even be overweight.

In fact, malnutrition could be one of the main reasons why many people are overweight. They may be eating too many empty calories and not enough food the body can use. The body, in its deepest inner wisdom, may know that it is missing some essential nutrients. It sends messages to the appropriate parts of the brain, setting up hunger and craving, despite plenty of calories already eaten, in the hope of getting the missing nutrients. Pregnant women commonly seem to experience this.

A doctor's physical exam can sometimes reveal signs of mild malnutrition, but it takes a sharp-eyed practitioner to spot them. Malnutrition can be assessed through a variety of tests, most of which are fairly expensive. However, a nutritionist's food frequency survey can be done as a relatively straightforward, inexpensive measure. It involves filling out a questionnaire in which the patient lists everything eaten over the past or several days. Not all doctors' offices would have these forms, but they are easily obtained from a nutritionist.

Alternatively, if you are not already taking a multivitamin, multimineral combination, start to take one. If you are already taking a multivitamin but are still feeling fatigued, consider switching brands. If this simple change does not result in your feeling better in a few weeks, you may want to seek additional nutritional advice (see Step 8). Many practitioners will provide guidance in detail, carefully diagnosing and treating a variety of nutrient deficiencies.

Toxicity

Just as common as malnutrition is the related issue of toxicity. Much of our food, air, and water is laden with chemicals that are metabolic monkey wrenches, making our metabolism function in a less than optimal fashion. Try for a couple of weeks to eat only natural whole foods, free of additives, preservatives, or other listed ingredients that you cannot pronounce. Try to avoid environments where you notice any fumes or chemical smells in the air. Also, for this trial period, drink only distilled water. Do all this for ten or fifteen days, and see if you feel more energetic.

For some people, toxicity is not simply mild and routine but is instead a severe specific exposure, perhaps on the job or at home. Rather than being a mild health irritation, a particular agent can be elevated to the category of a metabolic poison. It might need to be evaluated using special testing. Several people in our practice found that their low energy was caused by chlorine sensitivity. When they purchased shower filters and bottled water, their problems improved. For other people, it helped to eliminate certain industrial solvents or home-cleaning products.

Another consideration is the pollution of our air, water, and land from toxic waste substances that can permeate the water supply through leakage, including underground leaky gas tanks, ocean spills, and sewage leaks that may seem minuscule but can seriously confuse our immune systems. Pay attention to the health issues in your community, and begin to notice if there are unseen health challenges that need to be addressed. Many individuals in disadvantaged neighborhoods have toxic exposures due to nearby commercial facilities, including smokestacks on hospital incinerators and processing plants that use heavy industrial chemicals.

There are issues of environmental justice to be considered in the placement of these toxic facilities and dumps, which force some of our nation's poorest people, who are least able to speak out for themselves, to be exposed to substances that are very detrimental. It pays for all of us to help keep our communities safe by paying attention to water board reports and attending community forums addressing health and safety issues, especially those pertaining to the schools. Those who are most sensitive can often provide advance notice of future widespread havoc on public health by paying attention to their symptoms and by building support with others similarly challenged.

Fatigue Due to Lack of Exercise

Quite often a person can feel sluggish and have low stamina because he or she is not getting nearly enough physical activity. Most of the time, enjoyable exercise and exertion actually increase energy for the rest of the day. Although this is currently common knowledge, it is easy to forget when you are fatigued. Frequently, tired people feel they just don't have the energy to do any exercise at all.

To assess if you are a person who is fatigued because of insufficient exercise, force yourself to go for a brisk walk. If you feel better during, immediately after, or the day after exercise, then you are probably suffering from not getting enough exercise. If, on the other hand, you feel worse during, immediately after, or the day after exercise, you may well be suffering from low thyroid or a related condition. Feeling worse can be an indication that you were indeed "running nearly on empty," and now, after exercise, your gas tank is bone dry.

If it turns out that you are exercise-deficient, and you want to remedy the situation, start simply and cautiously. It can be very helpful to begin with deep breathing exercises to increase your cells' oxygenation and release of toxins. Drink plenty of water also. Then build your exercise program gently, proceeding with activities that appeal to you most. You may want to do power yoga but may need to build up to something this dramatic by first walking and practicing deep breathing. Then, as you find your body responding, you can move into aerobic and cardiac training exercises. The important thing is to pay attention to your body and work within its limits. If your body cannot handle exercise at all, you are in dire need of a good clinical evaluation. If you can exercise but still feel tired, you may want to consider a clinical trial of thyroid medication (see Step 5).

Allergy: A Common Energy Drain

Whenever people go to their health practitioner complaining of low energy, allergy should be a major consideration. Some people are mildly allergic to the same chemicals that cause severe chemical toxicity in others. These more mildly affected individuals are having an immune system response. Often the amount of chemical that would cause mild allergy is much, much less than the amount that would trigger a toxic response.

A complete blood count is, as we stated earlier, one of the simplest and least expensive of all blood tests. It is useful for determining who might have an allergy problem. A significantly high level of eosinophils could be an indicator that the low energy may be due to allergy. Other allergy blood tests can be ordered by a general practitioner, and allergy specialists can do even more detailed evaluations.

The simplest treatment for allergy is to avoid the allergen. If you can stop eating green beans (if you happen to be allergic to green beans), that will help tremendously. If you happen to be allergic to chocolate, it might be a bit harder to stop, but it would still be very useful to you. Many people eat chocolate daily, and find themselves getting more and more tired. Chocolate actually robs people of energy and is experienced as a major addiction for some folks, due to chemicals similar to caffeine, as well as its high level of magnesium. With increased magnesium intake, chocolate cravings often disappear.

If you are allergic to a particular kind of laundry detergent, dish soap, or bathroom cleaner, it would be a good idea to stop using that product. If, on the other hand, you are allergic to something that is not so easy to avoid, such as pollen, dust, or mold in the air, then you might benefit from being desensitized. This means going to an allergist and taking injections of diluted allergenic substances in order to desensitize the immune system to the allergen. Sometimes it is enough to take a symptom reliever, such as an antihistamine or over-the-counter homeopathic pills.

In addition, you can make simple dietary changes. If you are allergic to mold, keep in mind that the typical American diet contains large amounts of mold. A more optimal dietary choice for you may involve eating cottage cheese rather than aged cheese. Additionally, you may want to eat only fresh foods rather than leftovers, which grow mold even in the refrigerator. Beer and wine, which contain fermented products, may not be as good a choice as a mixed drink. Many people with mold sensitivities end up valuing their energy enough to live within these confines.

Some people who have allergies are tired because of an asthma-like lung response to the allergy. The lung problem results in less oxygen intake, and therefore decreased energy. A mild, undiagnosed asthma condition can result in less energy throughout the day and less comfortable sleep throughout the night. Proper interventions are essential. They can include natural remedies as well as prescription medicines. Definitely consult a specialist if you have any suspicion that your low energy may be due to allergic airway illness.

Our middle child spent weeks in bed during her junior year of high school, even with a treated thyroid condition, because she was mildly asthmatic and undiagnosed. When the asthma was treated, her entire energy profile changed dramatically, and she thrived in her senior year. (People who have low thyroid are much more likely to be bothered by their allergies and/or asthma than are people whose thyroid function is normal.)

Inflammatory Response: Another Energy Drain

Temporary low energy from a cold is one example of the brief fatigue caused by acute inflammation. Chronic inflammations, however, can be a major source of long-term energy drain.[1] These include chronic recurring sinus difficulty, chronic urinary tract infection, and chronic skin conditions. When mild, these generally do not affect overall energy level but instead are simply annoying. However, when they persist over a long period and become well established, they sap a person's overall energy for life. It is as if part of the body's vital force is depleted in constantly fighting the infection or holding it at bay.

Other less common chronic infections might involve the soft tissues of the musculoskeletal system, such as recurring tendinitis or bursitis. Chronic inflammation of the gastrointestinal tract may take the form of ileitis or colitis. These can be energy rip-offs, over and above the loss of energy they might cause because of the nutrient malabsorption.

A good internist can diagnose and treat these situations properly, while evaluating the possibility of coexistent low thyroid. A chronic infection is sometimes a symptom of low thyroid itself. Often when people are treated by specialists for these conditions, they obtain varying degrees of symptom control, but the root cause (undiagnosed low thyroid) is often left untreated.

For example, a dermatologist may prescribe pills and creams for chronic eczema, with 50 percent improvement of symptoms. If coexistent low thyroid is found and properly treated, symptom improvement may increase to 80 or 90 percent. Moreover, the person may feel better in general, in addition to the relief of the skin condition. Often people with low thyroid have a major irritating symptom, but also have several other minor symptoms that they did not know were related to a single underlying cause.

Lyme Disease

Lyme disease is a treatable, long-term infection that can cause low energy. It is caused by spirochete bacteria, which is carried by a few species of very small ticks. It can be hard to diagnose (tests are not totally reliable) and many people with chronic long-term fatigue actually are suffering from Lyme disease.

Not everyone with Lyme disease gets the characteristic "bull's-eye" rash. Some never see the tick or even know that they were bitten. Many people who are tentatively diagnosed as having other illnesses may in fact have Lyme, which can mimic various physical and psychological diseases. Lyme can cause a few additional symptoms that thyroid fatigue does not usually present, which include swelling and inflammation of the weight-bearing joints, as well as neurological problems. If you live in or have visited an area where you may have been exposed to Lyme disease, you should be fully evaluated to rule out this disorder.

Intestinal Parasites: An Emerging Problem?

For many years, a high incidence of parasitic disease was confined to third world countries. Things are quite different now. Changes in our ecosystem are affecting the industrialized nations. Heightened incidence of parasites could also be due to increased global travel, or to crowding as the result of population expansion. Whatever the cause may be, intestinal parasites are now quite common in this country among all classes of society. Part of the toll that they take is that they sap our vitality.

To make matters worse, most physicians don't even suspect this underlying condition. People can suffer for years with undiagnosed parasites. An intriguing wrinkle on the parasite problem is that their presence can irritate the immune system into making increased numbers of antibodies in an attempt to fight the foreign invader. The irritated immune system becomes overzealous, perhaps confused, and can start making antibodies against the body's glandular tissue. Can you guess which organ might be the most frequent target for this kind of mischief? If you guessed the thyroid gland, you are correct.

A person with this problem now has two reasons for low energy: the direct impact of the parasites themselves, and the indirect energy drain resulting from the autoimmune low thyroid response. As William Bendix used to say on *The Life of Riley,* a 1950s television show, "What a revolting development this is!" Fortunately, there is a simple, effective solution. If you suspect parasites, send a stool sample to a high-quality parasite laboratory (see Resources). If the results show the presence of treatable parasitic disease, then show the test to your doctor and get appropriate medication. Your thyroid will thank you.

Depression: A Common Cause of Low Energy

Depression is a major cause of low energy. Many people with depression suffer tremendous fatigue and a variety of physical symptoms. Depression is a serious medical condition, recently found to be neurological in nature. It involves depletion of the brain's neurotransmitters, chemicals that allow nerve transmission from one brain cell to another. Frequently a person who has low energy with no obvious cause is told that he or she must be depressed. This is a quick way of dismissing the problem and not doing any further investigation. Ironically, this diagnosis is frequently partially correct, because a person who has been suffering from low physical energy for extended periods can understandably feel a bit despondent about not being able to live life fully.

True clinical depression, however, is much more severe than the mild understandable depression seen in people as a side effect of being fatigued. Sometimes, treatment with antidepressants does not help at all, which makes one think that maybe the true diagnosis has been missed. Sometimes antidepressants work to a certain extent, but that does not rule out some other biochemical difficulty, such as low thyroid. Very frequently, in fact, low thyroid is a direct cause of depression. Studies at psychiatric clinics have found that many people seeking antidepressants for relief of depression actually had low thyroid as the cause of their symptoms.

Whatever the cause of the depression, it is important that it be treated properly. While many practitioners simply treat the symptoms, a good psychiatrist is well aware of the effects of borderline low thyroid on mood, and will treat both conditions accordingly.

Chronic Fatigue Syndrome: A Special Kind of Low Energy

When a person experiences severe and debilitating fatigue for over six months, not due to any of the situations discussed above, he or she may be suffering from the somewhat mysterious malady called chronic fatigue syndrome. There is a great deal of controversy regarding the existence of this syndrome, and even more controversy regarding its treatment. According to the researchers who believe that chronic fatigue syndrome is a definite disease entity, the correct term for the illness is chronic fatigue immune dysfunction syndrome

(CFIDS).[2] A significant number of people, especially in their twenties, thirties, and forties, seem to have this condition.

Researchers have isolated a number of immune system abnormalities, which describe a condition that is almost the reverse of AIDS. CFIDS has nothing to do with AIDS, the latter being a suppression of the immune system due to a virus's infecting the T-helper cells (these are the immune system's captains and lieutenants, organizing all the other immune cells). CFIDS, in contrast, appear to be characterized by an overactive immune system, one that is stuck in overdrive (some people even say stuck on red alert), and therefore becomes exhausted.

CFIDS is a particularly frustrating illness for the practitioner, because of the difficulty it poses in diagnosis, treatment, and management. However, it is a much more frustrating illness for the patient, who often finds that many practitioners do not even believe that the condition exists. These patients often feel doubly victimized, first by a baffling disease, then by a skeptical medical system that denies its reality.

Some people are convinced that they must have CFIDS, because other diagnoses have been ruled out. We find, however, that many of these people actually have undiagnosed low thyroid and not CFIDS. Low thyroid is easy to treat and has a very good prognosis for total recovery, compared to the much more complex treatment and much less rapid recovery required for people with CFIDS.

On the other hand, CFIDS and low thyroid often coexist. Doctors have long noticed that people with CFIDS commonly have elevated thyroid antibodies as part of the CFIDS overactive immune system. Treating the thyroid antibody elevation with the simple addition of thyroid hormone can often help the CFIDS condition.

Therefore, if you have CFIDS, you should be aware that in almost every chronic fatigue specialist's treatment protocol, there is an entry on treating the thyroid. This doesn't mean that low thyroid is the cause of your CFIDS. Rather, it means that treating the CFIDS with some thyroid hormone might be beneficial, especially when combined with other maneuvers that have been shown to be effective against CFIDS.

Hyperthyroidism

Sometimes, paradoxically, an elevated thyroid condition can cause low energy. Hyperthyroidism causes a person to be "tired and wired" for so long that eventually "tired" wins out, and the person becomes quite depleted. The diagnosis of high thyroid is generally easily made on physical examination and easily confirmed via blood tests. Hyperthyroidism is much less common than hypothyroidism, or low thyroid.

Stranger Than Fiction

Low thyroid can coexist with any of the other above low energy conditions. In fact, it can even coexist with high thyroid. This condition is called Hashitoxicosis, signifying the combination of the low thyroid component (Hashimoto's thyroiditis) with the high thyroid component (thyrotoxicosis).

Some people who have this rare condition complain of being exhausted yet feeling as if they are stuck in high gear. Others who have this malady feel high thyroid one day and low thyroid the next. It is as if a car is stuck in neutral, with the engine racing but with no movement. Some describe feeling as if there is one foot on the brake, the other on the gas. While diagnosis and treatment of Hashitoxicosis are complex, Japanese doctors have had some success using medications for both illnesses simultaneously.

Although few people have this condition, we wanted to mention it in order to emphasize that low energy isn't always what it appears to be. It may not fit the doctor's diagnostic model. For that reason, we believe strongly that the greatest test of all is to keep listening to your body, to pay attention to subtle cues and changes, and to have ongoing direct communication frequently with your practitioner.

This leads to an important final point. It is not simply that low thyroid can coexist with any of the above low energy conditions. Low thyroid can coexist with *any* condition. It can easily coexist with an unrelated serious illness. Low thyroid can work in the background of arthritis, diabetes, cancer, or heart disease. Untreated, it can make any of these serious illnesses even more severe.

In these concomitant situations, the low thyroid is not causing the more serious illness but is exaggerating the symptoms of the other illness. If the gas pedal in your car cannot be pushed down very far, then your car will not run very fast. If your thyroid is sluggish, then your regenerative and healing potential—for any health challenge—is diminished. Therefore, treatment of the low thyroid condition can result in improvements in overall health and even in the concomitant illnesses.

A Self-Assessment

Now it's time to determine if some undiagnosed low energy condition beyond low thyroid might be part of your health picture. In addition to having low energy and becoming easily fatigued, do you also experience:

- Dizziness or lack of balance, sometimes almost fainting or falling?

- Significantly disturbed vision or other neurological annoyances?
- A history of most of your symptoms having started suddenly at around the same time?
- Symptoms that are not at all relieved by extra rest or sleep?
- The pattern of "having to pay" (for previously tolerated exertion) for a whole day or two afterward?
- Some quite good days mixed with mostly bad days?
- The sensation that pressure at particular points on the body will trigger the whole area into major discomfort?
- Muscle spasms and gripping pain for no apparent reason?
- Bladder function that is severely erratic or irritable?
- Major sweating at night, or continual low-grade fever?
- What seems to be long-lasting inflammation/tenderness of lymph nodes in the neck, armpits, or groin?
- Severe sensitivity to particular foods, substances, or exposures?
- Recurrent inflammation or swelling of a weight-bearing joint?
- Immediate improvement with better food or vitamin intake?

A "yes" answer to four or more of these questions suggests that you may have something other than simple low thyroid causing or adding to your symptoms. Have a good practitioner check your situation carefully, conduct the necessary tests, and pinpoint the true source of your health issues.

The Bottom Line

- Low thyroid often coexists with other illnesses, sometimes partly causing them, sometimes caused by them.

- These other conditions can be common diagnoses like anemia or depression. On the other hand, they can be more unusual diagnoses like intestinal parasites or chronic fatigue immune dysfunction syndrome (CFIDS).
- Carefully evaluating and treating coexistent low thyroid is a crucial part of managing any illness, because undiagnosed low thyroid makes any other condition worse.

Use Signs, Symptoms, and Family History to Support a Diagnosis

The key to accurate diagnosis of thyroid disease is a high index of clinical suspicion.

—J. HERSHMAN, M.D., *Patient Care*

The Symptomatic Patient: How to Recognize Low Thyroid

Arriving late at our office, thirty-nine-year-old Regina looked burned out, a typical Silicon Valley casualty. Her problems were clear: "I feel constantly tired. I'm also a little disoriented, spacey, and kind of aching all over, especially in the head. My emotions seem off, but I don't want to take a pill to cover things over. None of this is very severe. I'm just mildly exhausted all the time. I'm even tired when I wake up from a good night's sleep. I've been to see an internist, a nutritionist, and a chiropractor. Everything seems to be normal. I even had a neurologic exam and an MRI of the brain—both normal."

It was true. A tremendous number of medical visits, workups, and lab tests had shown nothing. Regina felt like she was operating at 40 percent of her normal self, yet she was told by her doctors, "There doesn't seem to be anything that we can do." There appeared to be no explanation for her fatigue.

A very careful history, however, revealed additional noteworthy information: she had become increasingly slow in moving—even her bowels were sluggish. She had mild depression, her face turned red with exercise, and she had an occasional migraine along with regular headaches. In addition to all this, she had been increasingly overweight for the last several years, and had had no sex drive for the last six months. Her usually good memory was diminished, and her previously strong fingernails were now brittle and splitting.

Test results at our office were similar to the blood work obtained by every other doctor—totally normal. Physical exam was likewise normal. The only clue to her diagnosis was the particular constellation of symptoms outlined above. Based on her lethargy, mild depression, weight gain, loss of libido, and brittle fingernails, we started Regina on a clinical trial of thyroid pills.

Within three weeks, Regina felt quite a bit better. "I'm mentally more clear now. Even people at work notice they don't have to repeat themselves. I'm less disoriented, and more able to move and think faster, too. Best of all, I'm starting to feel better about myself. I definitely have more energy, and I'm happier now. I'm more comfortable in my body. There's less headache, and my constipation is totally gone. I'm telling you—it's a miracle!"

After three more weeks on thyroid medication, Regina reported feeling better than she had felt in years. She seemed like a different person.

The Thyroid "Low": A Special Fatigue

As Regina's story illustrates, a major hallmark of sluggish metabolism is fatigue, accompanied by other annoying symptoms. Generally speaking, the thyroid low is a fatigue that is not so bad in the morning, but gradually worsens over the course of a day. It can be a moderate tiredness that is somewhat refreshed by rest and sleep. On the other hand, it is sometimes a profound, bone-weary exhaustion that persists around the clock, day in and day out.[1]

As detailed in Step 2, although fatigue is a common main symptom for people with this disease, it is certainly not the only one. There is a long list of other possible major and minor clinical symptoms. Some people have only one symptom, while others have several.[2]

Additional Symptoms

June came to us with a visual problem. She had already been examined by an ophthalmologist who could find no reason for her complaint of "shaky" vision. A neurologist had found no brain tumor. She was then told that perhaps she needed a psychologist.

Ironically, June herself was a psychologist, as well as an exercise devotee. She felt healthy, both physically and mentally. She said to herself, "I don't need any psychotherapy. There's something wrong, and the internist can't find it."

After taking a detailed medical history, which revealed a few minor symptoms of borderline low metabolism, we suspected a possible thyroid problem, causing eye muscle fatigue. Through special blood testing, that suspicion was confirmed. When June was given thyroid medication, the eye problem went away.

June's case is an example of a person experiencing mainly one rather uncommon symptom of low thyroid. More often, people experience a collection of bothersome annoyances, with one main symptom predominating.[3]

Kirsten, a trim and healthy-looking forty-eight-year-old woman, consulted us about her severe eczema. The rash was persistent and aggravating, despite ten years of doctors' appointments and prescription medicines. Kirsten was generally fit, with her major problem being eczema extending over her thighs and buttocks. She had been treated by doctors in a major university medical center dermatology group, plus a homeopath and an acupuncturist. She had experimented with Chinese herbs, in addition to cortisone creams and pills. None of this was very helpful. She had suffered with this mild misery for almost a decade.

Close questioning of Kirsten regarding her medical history revealed additional clues: high cholesterol despite a good diet, occasional migraine headaches, a sense of fullness after eating, redness in the face with exercise, mildly cold hands and feet, moderately low sex drive, and mildly low red blood cells with normal serum iron levels. (Some people with normal amounts of iron are not able to use the iron to make red blood cells because their thyroid is low.) Her physical examination and test results were otherwise normal.

Because of this particular group of additional symptoms, we started Kirsten on thyroid hormone, beginning with a very small dose. She returned several weeks later reporting that her digestion was better and that her skin was beginning to clear. After a few more weeks, on a slightly higher dose, she was notably improved. The eczema was better than it had been in years. She had more energy, and her hands and feet were warmer.

On a full dose of thyroid medicine, after another month, Kirsten was dramatically improved. Her general energy was much better, she was feeling good, and her skin was now 90 percent improved. One month later, her skin was almost perfect, with no remaining rash. Her bloating was gone as well. This improvement has continued for years.

Kirsten went from wishing that the days would go by quickly, because she was in such discomfort, to wishing there were more time in each day. She wanted more time for watercolor classes, reading, writing, going on picnics, going to the lake with her family, wearing bathing suits, and pursuing the many other activities she had formerly avoided. She looked back in dismay to those days when she could do nothing about the severe eczema, other than to soothe it a bit with heavy applications of cortisone cream.

As you can see, people sometimes suffer needlessly for years from thyroid-related conditions. In addition to fatigue, vision problems, and troubled skin, there is a host of other additional symptoms of low thyroid. At the end of this step you'll find a self-assessment questionnaire that includes many of the difficulties that our patients have consistently reported. If you have several of the symptoms mentioned, you may wish to get your thyroid checked very carefully.

Thyroid disease can slow down every aspect of your life, including your mental and emotional well being, as well as a multitude of different body functions. This amazing diversity becomes more understandable when you remember that the thyroid gland is the throttle for every organ and cell in your body.

Related Conditions: Diagnoses That Increase Your Chances of Also Having Low Thyroid

If you cannot make a compelling case for low thyroid based on symptoms alone, you might want to ask yourself if you have one of the several thyroid-related conditions. These are not caused by low thyroid but often coexist with it.

For instance, you are more likely also to have a thyroid problem if you have anemia, vitiligo, Raynaud's syndrome, attention deficit disorder, alopecia, dyslexia, left-handedness (not an illness—just statistically relevant), rapid-cycling manic depression, mitral valve prolapse, carpal tunnel syndrome, Crohn's disease, ulcerative colitis, tendinitis, bursitis, or significant allergies. In addition, your likelihood of having low thyroid is greater if you have one of the autoimmune diseases, including diabetes, rheumatoid arthritis, lupus, sarcoidosis, scleroderma, myasthenia gravis, multiple sclerosis, thrombocytopenia, or Sjögren's syndrome.

Fred was an occasional tennis player with recurrent tennis elbow, a painful condition caused by inflammation of a tendon. Because of an undiagnosed low thyroid, however, this athletic twenty-six-year-old had a more enduring tendinitis that was more difficult to treat and harder to resolve. Since his overall curative force was diminished by sluggish metabolism, he just couldn't get rid of that tendinitis, despite assiduous use of heat, medication, physical therapy, and ultrasound. It wasn't until he finally received thyroid hormone that his body began to heal normally, and the condition resolved.

If low thyroid coexists with a major illness such as diabetes, you may then need a more aggressive treatment program, such as additional insulin or a stricter diet. Even so, these extra maneuvers may not accomplish the job fully. Your low thyroid makes all other body processes incredibly difficult to balance.[4] If your basic healing mechanisms are at a low ebb, they will not do their job well, even with outside assistance.

Consider the joint dysfunction experienced by David. His first onset of rheumatoid-like arthritis occurred ten years ago, when he was in professional school. He always thought it was somewhat psychological, saying, "I can't loosen up in this environment. It's stifling here."

Such was David's description of higher education, but the arthritis was real. It was treated by doctors using a variety of medications. We found that David also had high cholesterol, despite a healthy diet and optimal exercise. He was, in addition, mildly depressed. His skin was dry, and he was twenty pounds overweight. A half hour after eating any sweets, he would become distressingly sleepy. He often felt chilly, had a lower sex drive than usual (for him), had multiple allergies, and experienced bouts of memory loss.

David wanted a trial of thyroid hormone, partly because of his multiple symptoms, and partly because he had a friend who had improved as a result of taking it. Largely because arthritis is one of the associated illnesses of low thyroid, we started him on a small dose of thyroid hormone, while he continued to take medication for his arthritis. The initial small dose of thyroid medicine increased David's energy level only slightly. A larger dose seemed to work better. He now needed fewer anti-inflammatory pills, because his arthritis was improved. In addition, he had more energy in the afternoon, and was able to tolerate more exercise. We increased the thyroid dosage further, keeping a careful watch for possible side effects as the result of too large a dose. We will discuss these later on.

Since then David has been much less arthritic. He no longer

avoids taking hikes and has even been successful with slow jogging, which in the past had always made his knees and ankles worse. Overall he felt that he had 90 percent of his health back, compared to the 50 percent he started with. Treating his previously undiagnosed low thyroid condition was a big factor in improving his other physical conditions.

Family History: Is It in Your Genes?

Another tool to help diagnose low thyroid is family history. This term addresses illnesses you might have inherited. For instance, if your mother, sister, grandmother, or aunt had a thyroid problem, especially if more than one of them did, it is likely that you may develop a thyroid problem.[5]

Leona was a hefty high school physical education teacher referred to us by a chiropractor because her musculoskeletal manipulation therapy was not going well. The problem had begun three years ago, but had became much worse recently. Leona had always endured cold hands and feet, but this tendency also had worsened in the last few years. She also had become more tired and was starting to have phobias. She recently had developed increased pulse with mild exertion, a deepened sense of exhaustion, and feelings of severe anxiety. She was having heart palpitations and allergies, which she had never had before. At forty-one years of age, she found her periods becoming irregular, with a longer duration of PMS.

Leona had been given many of the thyroid tests. All had been normal. There was absolutely no indication of low metabolism, except that careful exploration of her family history revealed that her grandmother had suffered from a thyroid condition. Since no other cause of her severe symptoms could be found, we recommended that Leona try a course of thyroid hormone.

When she reported back to us a month later, she had more energy and was less tired and less depleted. It had taken only five days to notice some of these results. In ten days, her hands and feet were less cold, and a friend had noticed her improved color. Her chiropractor reported that her skin definitely felt warmer, and that the adjustments were now holding well.

All of this improvement, however, began to fade by the end of three more weeks. If she missed one day of her medicine, she felt miserable. We determined that Leona's setback was likely a result of too low a dose of medication. A higher dose brought back all the initial improvements. She also felt less panic, slept better, was more relaxed and had fewer heart palpitations. She was less sweaty at night, had decreased PMS, and could now stand up without becoming dizzy. Overall, the main improvement was her enhanced energy level. Leona and her entire family were delighted.

Maybe you can be delighted as well. Keep in mind that a thyroid problem in the family makes it much more likely that you could have a thyroid problem. How much more likely is it?

Take diabetes as an example of a strongly inherited illness. Most people realize that if you have a parent, sibling, or grandparent with diabetes, then it is important for you to be checked for diabetes yourself. Compared to diabetes, low thyroid has an even stronger hereditary component. With a family history indicative of low thyroid (or even highly suspicious for it), it is crucial to check yourself carefully for thyroid.

We see large numbers of people in our medical practice who have many symptoms for low thyroid, but whose tests do not show that they have the problem. In this situation, the positive family history is decisive, and the patient often benefits from a clinical trial of thyroid medication. Even the family trait of some members turning gray before the age of forty compels us to consider low thyroid.

At other medical practices, the scenario is often different. Symptomatic patients with normal tests are generally told they definitely do not have a thyroid problem. Then the patients say to the doctor, "But my mother had all of these symptoms, too. When she took thyroid hormone, she got much better. Her weight went down, her energy went up, and she got rid of a lot of her depression. She's doing really well now, playing golf and participating in volunteer activities. Now here I am, having similar symptoms starting at a similar age, and you're telling me I don't have a thyroid problem. Are you sure you've done the right tests?"

In such a situation, we believe that a clinical trial of thyroid hormone is indicated. Other doctors may not agree. In those instances, there is something else you might consider doing. Rather than switching doctors, you might instead ask for one or two special blood tests, as described in our next step. Also, some subtle signs may be evident on physical examination.

Physical Signs of Low Thyroid

There are a number of objective low thyroid *signs* that doctors can observe during the physical exam of the patient, and that others can notice as well. These differ from subjective *symptoms,* which are sensations verbally described by the patient.

These signs include:

Overall listless demeanor
Slow body movement and/or slow speech

Sluggish eye movements or slow pupil light reflex

Prominent bags under eyes

Abnormality in shape, size, consistency, or texture of thyroid
    gland

Difficulty in swallowing on command

Cool skin, as well as low oral temperature

Skin that is excessively dry or rough

Water retention, especially in the area of the face

Slow pulse

Low blood pressure

Hard-to-elicit or slow-moving ankle reflexes

Loss of the outer one-third of eyebrows

Unfortunately, it does not usually matter how many of these
physical signs are found during the exam: If subsequent blood tests
are normal, doctors seldom make a diagnosis of low thyroid. Step 4
describes what one can do in this situation.

The Basal Temperature Test: Another Simple Tool

Body temperature might be one of the most useful of all signs that
can be observed by the physician—or by the patient. Since the thyroid gland controls our metabolism, one simple measure of metabolic
rate is body temperature. As the famous thyroid doctor Broda Barnes
wrote in *Hypothyroidism: The Unsuspected Illness*, "More information
can be brought to the physician with only the aid of an ordinary thermometer, than can be attained with all other thyroid function tests
combined."

Some people run a higher basal temperature than others, but in
general there is a certain range that is considered desirable. If your

basal temperature falls well below that range, you may be dealing with sluggish metabolism.

The goal of this thermometer test is to measure your body's temperature while you are sleeping, or nearly sleeping, to determine how low your metabolism actually is. One of the best ways to approximate this is to measure your basal temperature when you first awaken in the morning. This means that you measure your basal temperature before you get out of bed or even sit up. You do it while you're still lying down, quite calm and peaceful.

The procedure itself is best done using a special thermometer called a mercury basal thermometer, available at most drug stores, which is calibrated for small temperature changes in and around the normal range. Many women use it to determine when they are ovulating.

Because a woman's basal temperature fluctuates as a normal part of her menstrual cycle, she should do this test during the first few days after her period starts. Men can measure their basal temperature at any time of the month. The mercury bulb of the thermometer is placed in the center of the bare armpit, and the arm then is returned to normal position, comfortably resting at the side of the body. The underarm temperature is a little more accurate for this purpose than the under-the-tongue method.

To arrive at your basal temperature, take your morning temperature for several days in a row, and then average the findings. Your average temperature should be close to 98 degrees. While "normal" varies quite a bit, if you are a whole degree or more below this range, you could have sluggish metabolism, especially if you have other signs and symptoms.

The basal temperature test might be as useful as many of the tests previously described. It is certainly much less expensive and less invasive than other tests. It is an example of what we call "appropriate technology" in health care: a simple, low-cost, consumer-controlled maneuver that might well be as useful as the higher-tech, higher-priced, more invasive options.

However, even the basal temperature determination is still just one test. This particular method of measuring your temperature is fraught with difficulties and inaccuracies, so it is best to do this test for many days in a row. Thermometers are notoriously inaccurate. You can increase the accuracy of the test by repeating the test later with a different thermometer.

This temperature test is not part of what is considered the standard diagnosis of low thyroid. Nevertheless, if you consistently get a reading that is well below the normal range, then you may want to consider yourself as someone suffering from sluggish metabolism. Consistently low temperatures, especially in someone who has some of the other symptoms and a family history of thyroid, can be quite compelling.

Although evaluation of symptoms, related illnesses, family history, and physical signs can offer a more thorough determination of your likelihood of having low thyroid, the proof is often revealed in how you feel once you take corrective measures. Some low thyroid sufferers have just one symptom or physical sign, with no other findings. If their persistent difficulty is truly due to low thyroid, they will often benefit greatly from treatment. For this reason, out motto has become "How you feel is the greatest test of all."

A Self-Assessment

The following is a list of symptoms, conditions, and signs that could be indicators of low thyroid. Take this self-assessment to see if you should receive further testing, or a trial of thyroid hormone, regardless of test results.

1. *Additional Symptoms*

Do you have:

- **Significant fatigue, lethargy, sluggishness**
- hoarseness for no particular reason
- chronic recurrent infection(s)
- decreased sweating even with mild exercise
- depression, to the point of being a bothersome problem
- a tendency to be slow to heat up, even in a sauna
- constipation despite adequate fiber and liquids in diet
- brittle nails that crack or peel easily
- high cholesterol despite good diet
- frequent headaches (especially migraine)
- irregular menstruation, severe PMS, ovarian cysts, or endometriosis
- unusually low sex drive
- red face with exercise
- accelerated worsening of eyesight or hearing
- palpitations or uncomfortably noticeable heartbeat
- difficulty in drawing a full breath, for no apparent reason
- mood swings, especially anxiety, panic, or phobia
- gum problems
- mild choking sensation or difficulty swallowing
- excessive menopause symptoms, not well relieved with estrogen
- major weight gain
- aches and pains of limbs, unrelated to exertion
- skin problems of adult acne, eczema, or severe dry skin

- vague and mildly annoying chest discomfort, unrelated to exercise
- feeling off balance
- infertility
- annoying burning or tingling sensations that come and go
- the experience of being colder than other people around you
- difficulty maintaining standard weight with a sensible food intake
- problems with memory, focus, or concentration
- more than normal amounts of hair come out in the brush or shower
- difficulty maintaining stamina throughout the day

2. *Related Conditions*
Have you ever had:

- **any of these autoimmune disorders: diabetes, rheumatoid arthritis, lupus, sarcoidosis, scleroderma, Sjögren's syndrome, biliary cirrhosis, myasthenia gravis, multiple sclerosis, Crohn's disease, ulcerative colitis, thrombocytopenia (decreased blood platelets)**
- prematurely gray hair
- anemia, especially the B_{12} deficiency type
- dyslexia
- persistent unusual visual changes
- rapid cycle bipolar disorder (manic-depressive illness)
- Raynaud's syndrome (white or blue discoloration of fingers or toes when cold)
- mitral valve prolapse

- carpal tunnel syndrome
- persistent tendinitis or bursitis
- atrial fibrillation
- alopecia (losing hair, especially in discrete patches)
- calcium deficiency
- attention deficit disorder (ADD)
- vitiligo (persistent large white patches on skin)
- neck injury, such as whiplash or blunt trauma

3. *Family History*

Have any of your blood relatives ever had:

- **high or low thyroid, or thyroid goiter**
- prematurely gray hair
- complete or partial left-handedness
- diabetes
- rheumatoid arthritis
- lupus
- sarcoidosis
- scleroderma
- Sjögren's syndrome
- biliary cirrhosis
- myasthenia gravis
- multiple sclerosis
- Crohn's disease
- ulcerative colitis
- thrombocytopenia (decreased blood platelets)

4. *Physical Signs*

Have you or your doctor observed any of the following:

- **low basal temperature in early morning (average of less than 97.6 degrees over 7 days)**
- slow movements, slow speech, slow reaction time
- muscle weakness
- thick tongue (seemingly too big for mouth)
- swelling of feet
- swelling of eyelids or bags under eyes
- decreased color of lips or yellowing of skin
- swelling at base of neck (enlarged thyroid gland)
- asymmetry, lumpiness, or other irregularity of thyroid gland
- swelling of face
- excess ear wax
- dry mouth and/or dry eyes
- noticeably cool skin
- excessively dry or excessively coarse skin
- especially low blood pressure
- decreased ankle reflexes or normal reflexes with slow recovery phase
- noticeably slow pulse rate without having exercised regularly
- loss of outer one-third of eyebrows

Scoring Your Self Assessment

FOR CATEGORY 1: ADDITIONAL SYMPTOMS

Give yourself 5 points for significant fatigue, and one point for each additional "yes" answer.

For Category 2: Related Conditions

Give yourself 5 points for autoimmune illness, and one point for each additional "yes" answer.

For Category 3: Family History

Give yourself 5 points for blood relatives ever having a thyroid problem, and 1 point for each additional "yes" answer.

For Category 4: Physical Signs

Give yourself 5 points for low basal temperature, and 1 point for each additional "yes" answer.

Interpreting Your Point Score

Add up your grand total of points from all four categories above.

- **5 points** = only mildly indicative of low thyroid
  Possible action: follow conservative suggestions in Step 8 for care and feeding of the thyroid gland.
- **10 points** = somewhat suspicious for low thyroid
  Possible action: obtain TSH level as first screening test
- **15 points** = very suspicious for low thyroid
  Possible action: obtain additional tests, if TSH is normal
- **20 points** = likely to be low thyroid
  Possible action: obtain all possible blood testing to help confirm a diagnosis
- **25 or more** = very likely to be low thyroid
  Possible action: obtain a trial of thyroid medicine, regardless of blood test results.[6]

Realize You May Still Be Low Thyroid Despite Normal Tests

Thyroid tests do not replace good clinical judgment, and should not be used alone to confirm or refute a diagnostic impression, or to dictate therapy.

—ERNEST MAZZAFERRI M.D., *Journal of Postgraduate Medicine*

As you learned from reading the previous step, the issue of blood testing warrants a very careful exploration. The decision to give or withhold thyroid medicine is currently based on "the tyranny of the test." Because of this powerful bias, many people are not receiving proper diagnosis or treatment. Here is the truth about thyroid blood tests: they are not as good as they need to be.

Patients who are sick with low thyroid find it very difficult to understand why their doctors aren't more aware of and sympathetic to their plight. They often have an emotional reaction, feeling discounted and oppressed when their condition is minimized. We hope that the following thyroid test information will assist you in asking the right questions of your health care providers.

Blood Testing: How to Know What to Ask For

This section provides a quick overview of the blood tests widely used for thyroid evaluation. You might consider discussing this part of the book with your physician (also see: "Show This to Your Doctor," page 261).

Why One Test Alone Is Not Always Sufficient

A thyroid blood test is the method used by most doctors to diagnose low thyroid. Any single test, however, cannot give the whole picture. Contrary to how most doctors evaluate it, the thyroid system is very complex. Looking at any one single test is akin to looking at a house you'd like to purchase through one window. Each test measures only one aspect of a much larger whole. Another aspect, perhaps the one that is not measured, may be the weak link in the chain of chemical reactions necessary for thyroid health.

If the one screening test performed on a patient with several thyroid symptoms turns out to be normal, additional tests should be ordered. Many low-thyroid patients, therefore, need to have several tests in order to be diagnosed correctly. Frequently, a correct diagnosis is missed, because people are given only one test instead of a whole panel.

Sometimes, the only test given is the T-4 (thyroxine) level. For years, the T-4 was considered the main indicator of whether your thyroid was high, low, or normal. The problem is that some people have a normal T-4 test, but are not doing well in terms of energy (their T-4 thyroid hormone level is normal, but not enough of it is being converted to active T-3 thyroid, which provides energy for life). This older screening test is not as revealing as more recently developed tests specifically for T-3 levels. If the T-4 test alone is within range, the doctor then says, "Your test is normal. I don't think you have low thyroid." The patient says, "Yes, but I still think I do."

Sometimes this impasse can be alleviated. Instead of just a T-4 test, or even the newly developed Free T-4 test (described below), the doctor can order what is commonly considered a basic thyroid panel, which includes a T-3U (T-3 resin uptake test) and FTI (free thyroxine index) added to the T-4 test. These additional two tests are an inexpensive attempt to determine if the levels of thyroid hormones, and the amount of thyroid-hormone binding protein in the bloodstream, are each adequate.

The thyroid panel sounds good, but we have found it to be only slightly better than the T-4 test alone in diagnosing low thyroid. In our experience, even more testing is often needed to provide a complete picture of thyroid function in mild hypothyroidism. In addition to the T-4, T-3U, and FTI, we add a TSH (thyroid stimulating hormone test).

TSH is the messenger chemical that instructs the thyroid gland to increase production of T-4 thyroid hormone (thyroxine). The TSH test thus measures the brain and pituitary's satisfaction with the amount of thyroid hormone in the bloodstream. A high level of TSH means that the brain and pituitary are asking for more thyroid hormone.

Jack's Story: One Missing Clue

Jack was a thirty-six-year-old whose chief complaint was "Something abnormal is causing me to overeat." Healthy as a kid, he was overweight as a five-foot eight-inch adult of 215 pounds. By going to Overeaters Anonymous and a nutritionist, he could hover at 195 pounds, but he still felt plagued by food cravings.

Jack also had severe fatigue, headaches, caffeine cravings, muscle tightness, excess gas, and weak ankles with several prior sprains. He had been given the basic thyroid panel (T-4, T-3U, FTI) by another doctor who had found that the results were within range and told him that his thyroid was fine.

At our office, he additionally received a TSH test. The result was definitely abnormal, indicating that Jack's monitoring systems (his brain and pituitary gland) were unsatisfied with the amount of thyroid hormone in his bloodstream, even though the basic thyroid panel had shown that amount to be within normal range. Jack was put on thyroid hormone replacement. After the very first pill, he noticed increased energy. After several days, he wasn't nearly as fatigued as he had been. When he gradually increased his dose, he found that it alleviated his headaches and muscle tightness.

After several more weeks, he felt more mentally alert, no longer dozing off in his afternoon meetings. He had much less intestinal gas. He felt a definite increase in ankle strength. But mainly, he experienced less preoccupation with food. He did not have nearly as many cravings, and he began to lose weight steadily. This was a tremendous improvement, especially for someone whose thyroid initially had tested out as "fine."

Jack's case shows why adding a TSH to the basic panel is a very good idea.[1] But what if the basic panel and the TSH are both normal? What if, as is the current trend, only TSH is tested, and it turns out normal? Despite the extra sensitivity of our new TSH tests, a mildly low-thyroid person can still appear normal on paper. We have found that people can easily have a sluggish metabolism and a normal TSH test (even if your doctor is using the highly or ultrasensitive version of this test).

A Key Piece of the Puzzle

The Total T-3 test is newer than the T-3U but older than the Free T-3 test. It may be better than either. The Total T-3, in our experience, is often quite useful in diagnosing low thyroid. It measures the total amount of fast-acting thyroid hormone in the bloodstream. The following is an example.

Justine had a long history of very good health prior to the onset of severe fatigue at age thirty-two. Significantly, this fatigue was accompanied by anxiety that was severe enough to prompt an evaluation by a psychiatrist. Although Justine needed to resolve a number of important family problems, the psychiatrist was well aware of the possibility of underlying medical conditions contributing to Justine's symptoms. He said, "You know, you're having more anxiety than any of this should cause. You seem to be a well-adjusted person overall. Why not get your thyroid checked?"

Justine went to her HMO doctor, who ordered the standard panel of the T-4, T-3U and FTI, as well as the TSH. All results were normal. There was no family history of low thyroid, and no associated illnesses. She was told unequivocally, "You do not have a thyroid problem."

When she asked us for a second opinion, we said we could certainly do a few more tests. The total T-3 came back low—not simply borderline low but very low! When Justine was given thyroid hormone, her symptoms of fatigue and anxiety completely disappeared.

We have used the total T-3 to diagnose a number of otherwise hidden thyroid problems. The total T-3 may be abnormal even when TSH is within normal range. A Total T-3 test can occasionally be abnormal for nonthyroid reasons, such as pneumonia or some other acute illness. This does not negate its usefulness in nonacute situations where people have chronic low-thyroid symptoms, such as Justine's.

Likewise, the newer Free T-3, in our opinion, also may be useful in uncovering borderline low thyroid in symptomatic patients, even when TSH is normal. The Free T-3 is a measure of the active thyroid hormone not bound to the blood transport proteins. Instead it is free to immediately enter into the cells. Similarly, a Free T-4 test measures the amount of thyroxine not bound to blood transport proteins and free to enter the cells.

The Last Straw

Finally, and of utmost importance, is testing for thyroid antibodies to ascertain whether the immune system may be sending out antibodies against the thyroid gland as if it were a foreign invader. A simple blood test can measure the amount of circulating thyroid antibodies being manufactured by the immune system. As discussed in Step 1, most low thyroid situations are autoimmune in nature and can be insidious.

All of the tests mentioned so far have been measures of hormone levels. Their outcome can be normal, yet the person can still be suffering from a thyroid condition. In certain instances, the only clue to the proper diagnosis is abnormal levels of antibodies directed against the thyroid gland. These are called antithyroid antibodies, thyroid autoantibodies, or simply thyroid antibodies. Whatever they are called, if they show up on blood testing, then you might have a mild thyroid problem, even though your hormone levels are perfect.

There are two main antibody tests, each designed to detect the presence of a specific thyroid antibody. One is called Antimicrosomal Antibody, more recently called Thyroid Peroxidase. The other is called Antithyroglobulin Antibody. In some people high levels of one or the other of these antibodies may be the only clue to their condition.

Many physicians think, however, that if all your regular thyroid tests are normal and the only elevation is in the antibodies, then you do not really have a thyroid problem. The controversy centers on the fact that a small percentage of completely healthy people, with no particular symptoms, have detectable levels of thyroid antibodies. We are not talking about these people in this book. A larger percentage of people have thyroid antibodies, are indeed symptomatic, and deserve proper treatment. At our clinic, we have seen many sluggish low thyroid individuals whose antibodies were the only telltale clue.

So, if you are bothered by low thyroid symptoms, but have normal results for your standard thyroid tests, you might want to ask for a test of your thyroid antibodies. It is a simple blood test, no more complicated than the others, even though doctors do not order it very often. It can be done at the same time as your other blood tests, or it can be done separately. We believe very strongly that if your thyroid antibodies are abnormal, and you have several of the symptoms associated with low thyroid, then you deserve the chance of a clinical trial of thyroid medicine.

Consider the following case: Celia, a twenty-nine-year-old, had been to seven doctors in the last two years for treatment of persistent herpes and various body pains. She also reported myriad other symptoms, which included depression, anxiety, and feeling chilly. Her main complaint was that she had occasionally felt tremendous fatigue, almost as if she were dying. From time to time, these brief episodes of low energy would prevent her from even rising from a chair. They were now occurring once or twice a week, understandably scaring her, since she had previously been in good health most of her life.

No one had been able to give her a diagnosis. She had been checked numerous times and was told all exams, procedures, and tests were normal. Her standard thyroid panel was normal. Even the TSH and Total T-3 were within normal range. This was a more complete thyroid panel than most people get, but it was still not adequate to pinpoint Celia's problem.

At our office, she was given the additional test of thyroid antibodies. In fact, in her case we used a very sensitive antibody determination using fluorescent antibody microsphere absorption (the FAMA Panel from IDL Lab—see Resources). This test showed significantly elevated antibody levels, indicating that thyroid disease might be involved.

She was given Synthroid 100 micrograms to start and told to return in three weeks. At that time, she reported that she had more energy for the day, much better sleep, and felt less foggy and thick-headed. She had more stamina, was less depressed and less chilly, and her aches and pains were diminished.

Her dosage was increased to 112 micrograms, which resulted in even more improvement by her third appointment. She no longer experienced any "bad pain days," could easily make it through a whole work shift, and was able to clean the house for the first time in years. Finally, she was sleeping well. She was able to deal comfortably with challenges, both at home and at work. Mainly, she was able to handle the kids without yelling and screaming or becoming overwhelmed. She finally felt free of depression. Over the course of a few months, she gradually became better. She felt more energy, less pain, and had fewer anxiety attacks. Happily, the herpes was much reduced as well. Her improvement was tremendous. We all began to realize how important this thyroid antibody factor had been in her overall health. Correcting it was not the solution to all of her problems, but it was certainly a major improvement.

One might ask why testing of antibodies is not done more often. We do not know. We believe that it should be a routine part of retesting whenever low thyroid is strongly suspected but the initial TSH test is normal. Very high levels of antibody do not necessarily mean a very severe state of thyroid illness. You might have a severe thyroid condition, with low levels of antibodies. In fact, you might have a severe version of autoimmune thyroid illness and have no antibodies show up at all. This is one reason why proper evaluation can be so elusive.

A good example is Judy, who had been evaluated by clinicians at the nearby university medical center. She had no family history of low thyroid, and no associated illnesses. She had a distressing number of symptoms, but all of her blood tests, including the antibodies, were normal.

She had even undergone a thyroid scan. This is an imaging technique that can reveal abnormalities of glandular structure. Judy's scan had been totally normal (see our discussion below of this and other special tests). In addition, she had been given an ultrasound evaluation, another imaging technique useful in revealing cysts, or enlargements of the thyroid tissue. Judy's ultrasound was also completely normal.

Judy was a nurse at a local hospital and had seen enough of this illness to know what it looked like. She had read about it in medical textbooks and felt certain that she was suffering from it. Judy told her doctor, "Okay, we've done all of these tests, and they're all normal. I still think I have thyroiditis. There must be some other way to confirm it."

Her doctor explained to her that the only further evaluation he could think of would be a cytology or cell evaluation. "We could remove a sample of the gland through a needle inserted in your neck and analyze it under the microscope. That's probably the only other thing that we can do." The doctor was sure that Judy would not be interested in this invasive procedure.

"Do it," Judy said emphatically, pointing to her neck. A needle aspiration cytology evaluation resulted in the unmistakable diagnosis of Hashimoto's autoimmune thyroiditis, moderate to severe. A standard dose of thyroid medication soon had Judy feeling better, despite the fact that her endocrinologist had, at first, sworn up and down that Judy did not have a thyroid problem.

Blood tests are simply one of several useful tools used in diagnosing thyroid problems.[2] Many other tools exist to support the diagnosis, as we discussed in Step 3. How could these often inaccurate blood tests have reached their present state of preeminence?

The Tyranny of the Test: Origins of a Dilemma

Why is there such "tyranny of the blood tests"? Why do so many people who need thyroid hormone not receive it? We believe there are several reasons.

The Attitudinal Challenge

Many physicians do not seem to be aware of the excessive prevalence of low thyroid in the population, or of its collective toll on the nation's health. As we have noted, investigations by university medical centers, as well as by the Mayo Clinic, have determined that the prevalence of this condition is quite high—compromising the health of as much as 10 percent of the population—and appears to be very much on the increase. It has taken a long time for the medical community, which is largely focused on critical care, to become aware of this dramatic situation.

Since the condition is usually not severe and certainly not life threatening, it may simply not grab the attention of busy doctors. Also, since the thyroid system controls so many aspects of physical and mental functioning, the patients' long list of complaints can seem unrelated and excessive to the clinician. The patient may have a skin problem, a stomach problem, feel chilly some of the time, and hot at others.

When confronted with this seemingly global array of symptoms, the physician is often skeptical and, rather than suspecting low thyroid, may believe that this patient may have a psychiatric problem. It is true that many thyroid sufferers are extremely sensitive and are aware of myriad diverse symptoms that are puzzling to them and their practitioners. The well-respected physician, J. Hershman, M.D., said it well: "The key to accurate diagnosis of thyroid disease is clinical suspicion of subtle signs."[3] We believe that the very subtlety and variety of symptoms reported by the patient should serve as a cue to physicians that the small but powerful thyroid might be the culprit.

When laboratory evaluation of the thyroid is requested, often only one test is ordered, the TSH. (Further explanation of TSH testing follows later in this step.) It is easy to add this test to a standard panel of blood determinations usually performed as part of a routine checkup (these include red and white cell counts, chemistries, and urinalysis). We reiterate that the TSH test alone is not always adequate.[4]

Suppose the TSH comes back normal. The doctor has fulfilled his or her responsibility, but the patient may be unhappy, and rightly so. As we said in Step 3, the TSH test may show little about the level of T-3 thyroid hormone or little about the presence of disturbingly high levels of thyroid antibodies. Unless additional tests are ordered, the

thyroid component of the patient's health problems may go unde-
tected. However, additional tests are expensive, and clinicians may be
reluctant to order them.

The Economic Challenge

There is a big economic factor related to blood tests for thyroid problems. The laboratory must make a determination of the level of a
complex molecule rather than a simple element, such as sodium or
potassium. Hormone levels are not easy to assess; consequently, testing for them is more costly. Testing for thyroid antibodies is even
more expensive and difficult than testing for thyroid hormone.

The expense of extra testing is minuscule, however, compared to
the enormous expense of evaluating and treating each of a patient's
multiple thyroid symptoms. Consider the expenses incurred when a
patient is treated by a dermatologist for chronic eczema, a gastroen-
terologist for irritable bowel syndrome, a neurologist for recurrent
migraines, and a rheumatologist for significant arthritis-like aches
and pains.

The expense of seeing multiple specialists, with their various diagnostic tests and procedures, dwarfs the cost of a full thyroid panel and
inexpensive thyroid hormone. Insurance companies, rightly concerned about the high cost of medical tests, may reason that "one
simple test will suffice." However, they may be operating from a perspective that is penny wise and pound foolish.

The Scientific Challenge

Another aspect of the problem is that currently available thyroid tests,
including the ultrasensitive TSH test, are not as scientifically accurate
as they need to be. The words "sensitivity" and "specificity" are used
to describe the accuracy of tests. A red blood cell count is quite "sen-

sitive," in that it identifies most of the people who have the condition of anemia. It is also quite "specific," in that it shows abnormal only in cases where levels of red blood cells are actually abnormal. The next time you are told that your thyroid test shows you definitely don't have a thyroid condition and do not need medication, tell the practitioner that you know that these tests are not as high in sensitivity and specificity as red and white counts. The doctor will then understand that you, the informed patient, know that you could be low thyroid and still have a normal test result.

The "Normal Range" Problem

Who decides what "normal range" is, anyway? Normal ranges are determined by researchers, who administer the tests to thousands of "normal" subjects. However, if a significant percentage of the population that is considered "normal" actually has some degree of borderline low thyroid, then the ranges of normal are inaccurate. Instead, what you have is a range typical for a large number of people with untreated hypothyroidism.

A similar situation prevailed for many years with regard to testing of cholesterol. We were taught in our medical training that a blood level of cholesterol under 250 was normal. That was incorrect in the light of further evidence demonstrating significant increased risk of heart attack if one's cholesterol was above 200. The earlier number had been determined as "normal" because it was very common to find men (women were not then considered to be as much at risk as they are today) with cholesterol levels between 200–250.

This is a risky range when compared to the average cholesterol level of the population of Japan, where there is a much lower incidence of heart disease. Thus, cholesterol in the range of 200–250 is normal only in a population of people who are prone to heart disease. Clearly, the normal range is not necessarily the optimal range.

The Evolution of Thyroid Testing

Let's take a closer look at these blood tests, this time through the lens of history. As long as low thyroid has been recognized as a disease entity, the tests for it have never been equal to the task of diagnosis. There have always been more people who had the condition than the tests could identify. Following is our version of modern medicine's search for an accurate thyroid test.

BMR Test

Fifty years ago, there was a test called the "BMR" (Basal Metabolic Rate), a time-consuming, laborious breathing test that was only partially accurate in differentiating who had low thyroid and who did not. It attempted to measure the amount of calories required to sustain the body's metabolic processes at rest. The methodology required the patient to breathe through a tube for several hours while lying completely still and it measured carbon dioxide excretion and oxygen consumption. At the time, it was the state of the art, although now it is considered quite crude.

PBI Test

The BMR was soon replaced by the PBI (Protein-Bound Iodine) test. The PBI measured the amount of iodine in the body that was bonded to protein carrier molecules. This test provided a rough estimate of the amount of T-3 and T-4 circulating in the bloodstream (recall that thyroid hormone is partly made of iodine, and travels in the bloodstream tightly bound to protein carrier molecules). No one would think of using a PBI test today because it was neither as sensitive nor as specific as was needed to diagnose the population accurately.

T-4 Testing: Direct Measurement of Thyroxine

Eventually, scientists learned how to measure thyroxine (T-4) directly from a blood sample. This became the new standard of excellence. It soon became clear, however, that thyroxine was not the active thyroid hormone in the body; it was thyronine (T-3). T-4 must first be converted into T-3.

The Thyroid Panel

Doctors were eventually able to measure the conversion of T-4 to T-3 indirectly by a test called T-3 Uptake, or T-3U. Then, a mathematical computation could be performed on the values for T-4 and T-3U. This new number was called the Free Thyroxine Index (FTI). It is an estimate of the amount of biologically active thyroid hormone in circulation. These three results, the T-4, T-3U, and FTI, came to constitute what is now called a thyroid panel. The currently used thyroid panel was much better at diagnosing low thyroid than the T-4 test alone. These days, however, it is considered by many to be inadequate.

TSH Test

The thyroid panel is not as sensitive and specific as a test for TSH (thyroid-stimulating hormone secreted from the pituitary gland). Recall that the brain controls the thyroid gland's production of thyroid hormone through the secretion of TSH from the pituitary gland.

The amount of TSH in the bloodstream is a useful indicator of whether one's thyroid gland is functioning in the extreme, either too high or too low. Because it can be used to diagnose both high and low thyroid, the TSH test has more recently been utilized by itself as the only thyroid test ordered for screening purposes. It may be the only test ordered, but it is not the only test needed, as you will see below.

We can recall when a TSH of 7.0 or below was considered normal. Years later, the TSH cutoff was 6.4, meaning that anything below that level was considered normal. Still later, the cutoff was moved to 5.5. Now, some labs are reporting a level of 4.2 as being the cutoff level, above which the patient may be hypothyroid.

This decrease in the TSH cutoff point seems significant to us. In fact, at our clinic, a TSH over 3 is considered suspicious, and anything over 4.0 merits treatment, if accompanied by other signs, symptoms, or family history.

Total T-3

Concurrent with the refinements in TSH testing, doctors started using a direct measurement of thyronine, called Total T-3 (the test is also called Total Triiodothyronine). In certain low or high thyroid patients, this test often showed abnormalities when the thyroid panel and the TSH were normal. We believe this was because the test measures the total amount of active thyroid hormone in the bloodstream. Nevertheless, some people were still undiagnosed, because even this test was insufficient.

Free T-4 and Free T-3

Almost all thyroid hormone in the bloodstream is tightly bound to blood carrier protein. In that form, it is not available to enter the cells. A small fraction, however, is free and ready to enter the cells immediately. Recently, it has become possible to measure the small fraction of Free T-3 and Free T-4. The Free T-3 and Free T-4 tests are helpful in determining who has low thyroid when other tests are normal. However, even these tests still do not identify all people who have a low thyroid condition.

TRH Test: The Present State of the Art?

The most sophisticated of all tests to reveal mild low thyroid is the TRH (Thyrotropin Releasing Hormone) test. TRH is secreted by a part of the brain called the hypothalamus. In contrast to the TSH test, which only measures the amount of thyroid stimulating hormone normally being released from the pituitary, the TRH test measures how much TSH the pituitary keeps in reserve.

With the TRH test, a more exquisitely sensitive analysis of the person's thyroid function can be made. The problem is that the TRH test requires an injection, followed by one or more blood draws (15, 30, and 45 minutes afterward). This is expensive and inconvenient for both patient and lab. Within the constraints of managed care medical plans, physicians order it less frequently than they did when private insurance was the norm. The TRH test is a useful test to obtain however, if you have symptoms of low thyroid or a family history of thyroid disease, with a "normal" TSH of 2.0 or above.

Lessons from the History of Thyroid Testing

You can see that there are many reasons for thyroid tests to be interpreted with a grain of salt. Until the "holy grail" of laboratory diagnosis of low thyroid has been discovered, there is no set of thyroid tests that will absolutely rule in or rule out the disease in all of the people tested for it. Perhaps the more expensive and more cumbersome TRH test could do this, but certainly not any single TSH test.

In these days when medical costs are high, the current trend is to do the TSH test alone. Nevertheless, we strongly maintain that no one test, or group of tests, should be used by doctors to state categorically, "You don't have low thyroid."

To further explain, let us draw on the doctor's "bible," the *Physicians' Desk Reference* (PDR).[5] In the Synthroid section, under the subheading "laboratory tests," physicians are advised not to rely solely on any one particular blood test for diagnosing and/or managing low thyroid. Instead, they are reminded to combine the knowledge obtained from laboratory evaluation with good clinical judgment. Yet, with managed care dictating protocol, physicians are by and large ignoring this advice.

Thus is derived what we have been calling "the tyranny of the test." Meanwhile, you deserve to receive proper treatment if you have the significant, yet hard-to-diagnose, medical condition called borderline low thyroid.

Beyond Diagnosis: How to Use the Tests for Optimal Thyroid Treatment

If the tests are not infallible for diagnosis, how good can they be for ongoing management of therapy? In certain other medical conditions, a different test is used for the ongoing monitoring of medication than the one used to diagnose the condition initially. For example, for many years, the test for *diagnosing* diabetes was a blood sugar level, drawn two hours after eating. The common test for *managing* diabetes was a fasting blood sugar level, drawn in the morning before breakfast.

In contrast, the tests used to manage a patient on thyroid treatment are the same tests that are used for the diagnosis of the condition. This may or may not be the best wisdom, but it is all we have presently.

Suppose a patient who is getting thyroid hormone treatment has a followup TSH test to determine the correctness of her dosage. Let's imagine that her original TSH was 6 on a normal range of 0.5–5.0. Now, the followup TSH test shows 3.8. A doctor might say, "This is perfect. Your TSH result is well within normal range. You are taking the right dose."

The patient, however, may feel only slightly better. She may have 30 percent improvement in only one symptom. The patient says, "Wait a minute. I'm not feeling that much better. How do we know this is my correct dose?" The doctor replies, "We know this is your correct dose because your TSH is in normal range now." This patient might experience much further improvement in several symptoms with more medicine, which may result in a lower but still normal TSH.

Some doctors prefer the lower limit of a corrected TSH to be 1.0. Others are comfortable with a TSH of 0.5. Some thyroid specialists at the University of California Medical Center in San Francisco like to see the corrected level around 0.2 (slightly below the normal range of 0.4–5.0). That figure is generally considered by many nonuniversity doctors to be too low, suggesting to them that the patient is on too much thyroid medication.

At our clinic, we have patients who do not feel well until they take enough medication to lower their TSH level to 0.1. However, that is a level that often makes medical practitioners uncomfortable. The stage is once again set for the tyranny of the test: The patient feels good, but only at a TSH level that feels bad to the doctor, based on the test.

Is Subnormal TSH a Desirable Treatment Goal?

Many researchers think that the stimulation of the thyroid gland by TSH results in a provocation of the antibody reaction, causing low thyroid. It can therefore be argued that people with autoimmune low thyroid do best with a very low TSH, indicating minimal stimulation of the thyroid gland. Having a TSH in the normal range may not be the right goal for optimum management of most low thyroid patients. Giving enough medicine to yield a subnormal TSH is called thyroid suppression therapy. We are convinced of its value in treating autoimmune low thyroid. The medical profession at large is still divided on this point.

In cases of symptom improvement only at lower-than-normal levels of TSH, it might be better for the doctor to follow the Total T-3, since this is a direct measure of active thyroid hormone. Why not track progress using the newer Free T-3 or Free T-4? These newer tests have been disappointing to us. We find they are frequently unrelated to patients' symptoms and physical findings. Once again, the newest tests may not be the best ones for you.

This doesn't mean that you should simply rely on the old tests. A professor of endocrinology once told us that when managing a known case of low thyroid, the T-4 level is the last thing you want to know. Why is that? Because sometimes a patient's T-4 level can rise slightly above normal on the proper dose of medication. Some patients don't feel decent until this happens, and if you measured their T-3 level, you would know why.

When such patients take standard doses of Synthroid, their T-4 level in the blood can be at the upper limit of normal, with the T-3 level still remaining too low for symptom relief. To get the more important number (T-3) into normal range, the less important number (T-4) has to be a bit high. Nonetheless, a slightly high T-4 makes many physicians uncomfortable, so their patients limp along with inadequate symptom relief.

The New Combined Approach

This imbalance between T-3 and T-4 is easily rectified in some patients by administering a mixture of T-3 and T-4, rather than following the common approach of using T-4 alone. Other patients do better when given Armour thyroid, which is a natural mix of T-3 and T-4. Be wary when a doctor tells you, "I know you are finally feeling good, but I have to lower your Synthroid. Your T-4 level is too high." At that point, you could say, "Why not do a total T-3 test, and perhaps add some T-3 to this lower Synthroid dose?"

Symptoms of excessive medication levels, whether T-3, T-4, or both, can include difficulty sleeping, feeling too hot, having a racing heartbeat, sweating for no reason, twitching muscles or tremor, rapid thoughts, and generally feeling too hyped up. If you have none of these symptoms, and you are finally feeling good, perhaps for the first time in years, you may not need to go down to a less satisfying dose. This is especially true if your doctor can find no signs of excess medication upon physical exam.

Sometimes this dosage dilemma can be a battle, because you are up against the tyranny of the test. Now, you can say to your doctor, "Listen, the goal of therapy is not to have a normal TSH or normal T-4. The goal of therapy is to have a normal patient. Can't you work with me on this?" Then show your doctor this book, or a similar one by endocrinology professor and thyroid journal editor Ridha Arem, M.D. (see Further Reading).

The Osteoporosis Debate

The scenario could continue as follows: "I understand that you're feeling better on the present amount of medicine, but as your doctor I have to warn you that you are risking osteoporosis as a result of this dose of thyroid medicine."

You've just been told that you are being a "bad" patient, because your desire for more medicine is going to hurt you in the future. The doctor has played his trump card, and you either cave in or learn more about osteoporosis.

This is a condition characterized by bone loss, especially from the hip and spine, with increased risk for fractures. Prevention of osteoporosis means keeping your bones strong.

Osteoporosis plagues our elderly population, causing anguish, expense, and perhaps early death. When an elderly person breaks a hip due to osteoporosis, severe depression or pneumonia may soon follow. Medical thinking about the effects of thyroid pills on bone density has been evolving.

The controversy started some years ago, when this research data was just beginning to be collected. The results suggested that thyroid hormone replacement was associated with a lowered bone density. Many doctors then became fearful of thyroxine and tried to treat hypothyroidism with as little medicine as possible. This resulted in many people receiving a dose too low to relieve their symptoms. It was considered a trade-off. Patients would have to continue suffering with some of the symptoms of their low thyroid now in order to preserve their bone density for the future.

However, the studies at that time lacked the data available today from third generation TSH assays and high-resolution bone densitometers. In addition, the groups of patients then being analyzed lacked the diversity necessary for accurate study. With further research studies pouring in, it now seems that thyroid medication— even in the higher doses that some people need to feel best—does not increase one's fracture risk in later years.

Careful research in the last few years reveals that appropriate doses of thyroid medication is not harmful to the bones of hypothyroid individuals. Multiple studies in the United States[6] and abroad[7] indicate that proper doses of medicine are *not* associated with increased fracture risk. This is fantastic news for millions of women! Contrary to what you are likely to be told, we now think that your greatest risk of osteoporosis might be from undiagnosed or undertreated hypothyroidism. You are definitely at risk for osteoporosis if you need thyroid hormone and do not take it. It is a medical fact that untreated low thyroid is a cause of osteoporosis.

There are many issues involved in maintaining a healthy bone density. For a review of this topic, we suggest you read the wonderful book *Preventing and Reversing Osteoporosis,* by Alan Gaby, M.D. (see Further Reading). Dr. Gaby contends that thyroid replacement therapy in appropriate doses does not harm the bones.

But what exactly is an appropriate dose? Depending upon how closely your doctor has followed this osteoporosis debate, you might get a very skewed opinion. Because most of the women in our family are on thyroid treatment, we have reviewed this literature very carefully. Our summary of the pros and cons boils down to this: find and stay on a type of thyroid that is good for you, at a dose that has you feeling your best. This is likely to be the best thing for your bones. In addition, do plenty of weight-bearing exercise, take 1,500–2,000 milligrams of calcium per day, and read what Alan Gaby, M.D, has to say on the subject. We also recommend progesterone cream and the excellent book about it by John Lee, M.D., *What Your Doctor May Not Tell You About Menopause* (see Further Reading).

Special Medical Tests and How They Can Help

Below are some highly sophisticated tests that can be useful in special circumstances. Most people with simple low thyroid do not need these types of tests.

Thyroid Scan

A thyroid scan is a picture of the gland taken after radioactive dye is injected into the body and concentrated in the thyroid area. This image reveals what the gland looks like and whether it is doing its job adequately.

How well the gland is doing is revealed by its uptake of the radioactive material. Severe high and low thyroid can show up on thyroid scans through high or low total uptake of the radioactive material.

Sometimes the scan will show that only one part of your thyroid gland is producing thyroid hormone. Occasionally, there are other abnormalities, and a scan can be very useful in pinpointing various rare, unusual conditions.

However, a scan is not very useful for diagnosing the routine, low thyroid conditions that we are discussing in this book. We have seen people with symptoms of low thyroid who feel much better on thyroid hormone, but whose scans appears fine, and whose uptakes are in the normal range.

A thyroid scan can be one further test that is more expensive, perhaps more risky, and certainly more invasive and time intensive than a simple blood test, and it may not show what you need to know.

Fine Needle Aspiration (FNA)

The FNA thyroid cytology (cell evaluation) test involves inserting a tiny needle into the gland and removing a small amount of tissue for laboratory analysis. It is generally reserved for patients who have a gland that is abnormal in appearance or feel, or whose scan shows a suspicious area. There might be enlargement, nodules, or abnormalities that need to be investigated in order to assess whether an enlarged area is harmlessly hollow (a benign fluid-filled cyst) or solid (such as a thyroid cancer tumor.)

A cytology evaluation is not needed often, but it can be very useful on certain occasions. If your problem is low thyroid, and your gland appears to be generally normal in size and shape, containing no particular lumps or bumps, an FNA is not at all indicated for you.

Thyroid Ultrasound

A much less invasive test than both thyroid scan and fine needle aspiration is the thyroid ultrasound. An ultrasound is more benign than a thyroid scan, in that radioactive material is not used. Instead, sound waves are sent into the neck and the echoes then measured, creating a picture of your thyroid that can show the presence of cysts in the gland, fluid-filled sacs, nodules, and other irregularities common to autoimmune thyroid. This information can be useful in diagnosing the more severe forms of the condition. However, you can have a normal thyroid ultrasound test and still have a low-functioning thyroid gland.

How You Can Escape the Tyranny of the Test

By this time, it must be abundantly clear that thyroid testing, *by itself,* should dictate neither thyroid diagnosis nor thyroid treatment. We hope that you will take the above suggestions to heart, and have fruitful discussions with the practitioners you choose.

Here are the final tips:

If your only thyroid test has been a T-4, or a T-4 panel, obtain a TSH level. If the TSH is normal, ask for other tests. Consider factors other than test results alone in making treatment decisions, and allow for other carefully considered sources of information to become part of the equation. New tools are being developed all the time, and some are easy to use and self-empowering. Thyroid function can be evaluated by saliva, urine, or electro-acupuncture, though these techniques are not currently accepted by the standard medical establishment (see Resources).

A weight-loss specialist, Sanford Siegal, D.O., M.D., has developed a four-week dietary test, based upon the fact that hypothyroidism causes a decrease in calories burned. His test measures this decrease in burned calories and helps to make a diagnosis when blood tests show nothing (see Resources).

The best way we know to diagnose and monitor low thyroid is by the thoughtful combination of medical history, physical exam, and a panel of tests, basal temperature being one of them. The blood tests, however, are still only part of the total picture. Only by pursuing multiple avenues of diagnosis can you overcome the tyranny of the blood test—and arrive at an accurate assessment.

The Bottom Line

- You could have low thyroid despite a normal TSH test.
- You could still be low thyroid despite any normal thyroid test.
- The above two situations may occur regardless of whether you are being diagnosed for the first time or are being checked after years of treatment.
- If your blood tests are normal, but you haven't been tested for thyroid antibodies, insist on this as a next step.
- Even more sensitive than TSH and antibody determinations is the TRH test.
- Most important, the greatest test of all is *how you feel*—and not a laboratory number.

Discover Your Best Dose, Brand, or Mix of Medicines

New data have forced a profound reassessment of long-held views of thyroid hormone production and have important clinical applications as well.

—MARK SCHIMMEL, M.D., *Annals of Internal Medicine*

How and Where to Begin

By this time, let us assume that you have learned about the connection between low thyroid and other fatigue-related illnesses, have made a provisional diagnosis, and understand more about testing dilemmas. You may now be ready to begin taking thyroid medication (if you are not already on it).

Often at this juncture new questions arise. What is the right medicine? What is the right dosage? In other words, how will you make decisions to ensure that you receive the optimal treatment?

The standard therapy for hypothyroidism is thyroxine, one of the two main thyroid hormones. It is synthesized in laboratories and is available in several different brands, the most well-known being Synthroid. Another name for thyroxine is T-4, also called slow-acting or storage thyroid hormone. T-4 must be converted in the body to thyronine (T-3), known as fast-acting, or active thyroid hormone. It, too, can be synthesized into pills, and its use in treatment will be described later in this step.

Most people are initially prescribed T-4. You can begin with a dose roughly equivalent to one microgram per pound of body weight, if you're not a very heavy person. In other words, a 125-pound person might be prescribed 125 micrograms of thyroxine as a starting dose; 125 micrograms (abbreviated as 125 mcg) is exactly the same dose as 0.125 milligrams (abbreviated as 0.125 mg). Thyroid doses are listed both ways.

The Ideal Program: A Gentle Start

Generally, it's a good idea to start slowly. A person who is prescribed 125 micrograms of thyroxine should start gradually, perhaps at 25 micrograms, for the first week, then 50 micrograms for the next week, then 75, then 100, and then 125 over the ensuing weeks. The body needs time to adjust to higher levels of this powerful hormone.

It may well be that you will feel some improvement at the very low dose of 25 micrograms. If so, you might want to stay at that dose for several weeks or more. When people notice improvement at low levels of medication, it shows how delightfully sensitive and responsive their bodies are to the new medication.

We recommend that you stay at a given dosage for as long as you continue to improve. You may stay at 25 micrograms for months, or even years, if that alone maintains sufficient improvement for you. However, this is not what usually occurs.

Instead, what is frequently observed is that the initial benefit—if any—of a small dose such as 25 micrograms begins to fade after a week or so. When that happens, it means that your body is ready for the next increment.

What happens more often, however, is that no initial improvement is seen at such a low dose. The desired improvement may not even be noticeable until you reach 50 or 100 micrograms. This improvement may last for weeks or months before it begins to wane. Once again, your body is telling you that it is ready for the next increment.

This process of gradually increasing dosage is called upper titration. If you do the titration with 25-microgram pills, at some point you will be taking five pills a day, for a total of 125 micrograms. These five pills are best taken all at once, in the morning. Later, if this turns out to be your correct level of medication, the low-dose pills can easily be converted to a single 125-microgram tablet. The new tablet will be the same size as the others, but it will be a different color, indicating its higher strength.

Some people do not want to take the time to start with a mild dose, adjusting to their medication gradually. However, we have found that the slow, step-by-step method of reaching your optimal dose is more easily tolerated by the body than the "sock it to me" approach so characteristic of our fast-paced culture.

You Might Need More Than the Standard Dose

Now suppose you're at 125 micrograms. It is possible that all you will ever need is this standard "rule of thumb" dosage. But suppose you begin to notice once again a waning of your sense of well-being. You might need more than one microgram of thyroxine per pound of body weight. If so, consider increasing your dosage to 137 or 150 micrograms, both of which are still in the range of standard dosage.

People who weigh more than 125 pounds might start their titration in a similar fashion, but their target dose may need to be a bit higher. For some reason, 150 micrograms is the highest dosage many doctors feel comfortable prescribing. We think, however, that such a dose may not allow you to achieve the comfort zone for your particular body. You might need to push for more, depending on your basal temperatures and test results, but especially depending upon your clinical response to the medicine. Many people who could do well on thyroxine do not find it very useful in relieving their symptoms, simply because they are not taking enough of it.

Suzanne, for example, came to our office a couple of years ago on her fiftieth birthday. Her appointment was part of her birthday present to herself. For a good part of the past five years she had been saying to herself, "I need to see someone else about my thyroid. I think I should be taking a higher dose." Suzanne had been taking 100 micrograms of Synthroid for twenty-two years. All had gone well until age forty-five, when she noticed the return of most of her original symptoms.

When she discussed this with her doctor at her yearly checkup, she received the typical response: "I can understand that you would like to take a higher dose, but your blood tests show that you're fine. Therefore, we're not going to increase your medicine at this time." On occasion, Suzanne had experimented by increasing the medicine herself, taking an extra half pill from time to time, with positive results. Yet even when she confronted her doctor with this bit of clinical information, the doctor refused to budge, saying, "Don't do that again. You must follow my dosage directions precisely. This is the best dose for you."

It seemed likely to us that the original dosage that had kept Suzanne quite healthy for many years was now too low. This can happen during periods of increased stress or major life changes. It can also occur after accidents, illness, or surgery. In Suzanne's case, the return of her symptoms seemed to be related to the onset of menopause.

The reason a person may need more thyroid hormone during stressful life events is twofold. First, it takes more energy to make a change than to maintain the status quo. Second, any stressful change can be easily interpreted by the immune system as a threat. As we have seen, increased immune activity in response to a perceived threat can be directed against the thyroid gland, resulting in decreased thyroid hormone output.

Upon physical exam, it was clear that Suzanne's symptoms were likely to be related to her hypothyroidism. Her blood pressure was 85/50, down from a normal level of 120/80. Her pulse was 50, and this low pulse was not the result of exercise (she did not have the strength to do any exercise at all). Her skin was markedly dry. Her reflexes were 1+ (on a scale of 1+ = too low, 2+ = just right, and 3+ = too high), and the recovery phase of her ankle reflex was quite sluggish, a cardinal sign of low thyroid. The blood tests that had been conducted by her regular doctor showed a TSH of 3. 7 (TSH normal is 0.5–5.0); T-4 of 6.1 (T-4 normal is 4.5–12); and a Total T-3 of 90 (Total T-3 normal 88–200 optimally, with anything under 100 possibly being suspicious).

Although Suzanne was well tested and well followed by her physician, he was not interpreting these tests as generously as we did. It appeared to us that she needed additional thyroid hormone, especially given that her total T-3 was under 100 and her TSH was not as low as we would like, although it was in the normal range.

When Suzanne's dosage of thyroxine was increased to 112 micrograms, she felt noticeably better within a week, but the improvement was not as great as when she had occasionally experimented with one and a half times her normal dosage for a whole week. One and a half of her old pills equaled 150 micrograms. She wanted to go straight to this dose. We reassured her that it might be better to work toward that dosage gradually and only as needed.

It turned out that 125 micrograms was better than 112, and 137 was better than 125. There was no additional benefit in going to 150. In fact, that dosage seemed to make her slightly agitated, so 137 was her final dose. The side effects of too much thyroid medicine feel similar to the effects of drinking too much coffee. They include: inability to concentrate, feelings of being jittery, hyped up and pressured, mild tremors, and a sense of being too warm. Occasionally there can also be a rapid heart rate or a sense of heart palpitation, and insomnia.

Lab tests at the dose of 137 showed a TSH of 0.2, T-4 of 10.8, and a Total T-3 of 132. These levels seemed preferable to us. Beyond that, Suzanne felt much improved. Once again, all her symptoms were relieved, and she felt like a new woman.

You Might Need Something Other Than Standard Medicine

A simple increase in thyroxine (T-4) made all the difference in Suzanne's case. Many others, however, do not have such good results with thyroxine, even though it is the most common of all the thyroid medicines used in this country.

Some people can begin to have difficulty with thyroxine after taking it successfully for many years. Others can have a problem with it after only a few weeks. Still others respond to it poorly from the very beginning, or experience no response at all. Sadly, if their blood tests look better than they did before treatment, their doctor may say, "Well, this is as good as you're going to do." We disagree.

There are numerous people with low thyroid who should be treated with something other than thyroxine (T-4). They might simply need a different brand of thyroxine, or perhaps thyroxine mixed with thyronine (T-3). It is even possible that a nonsynthetic, animal-derived thyroid medication, such as Armour thyroid, would be a more effective choice.

Consider first the problem of determining the exact brand of thyroxine that best answers your needs. There are currently three major brands of thyroxine sold in the United States:

Synthroid (the largest seller and one of the top most frequently
    prescribed drugs in America)
Levothroid
Levoxyl

These three different formulations of synthetic T-4 thyroid hormone are almost equivalent, but we have known many patients, as well as many doctors, who favor one over the other.

It's certainly understandable why a patient might have a favorite brand. Individual response to some of the pill's ingredients could easily result in a person doing slightly better with Levoxyl than with Synthroid. That same patient might also have a terrible time with Levothroid.

Often people come into our clinic saying, "Here's the brand that works best for me." We've seen this happen so many times that we tend to believe people when they say it. We think that they should have the brand that feels best for them, for whatever reason. We know of a number of doctors, not to mention entire HMOs, who have a "favorite" brand of thyroxine. However, it may not be your body's favorite brand. You may have to assert yourself to secure the right brand for you.

Did the Research Study Evaluate YOU?

Where does this brand bias come from? It may be related in part to the results of research studies, which are often funded by the company that stands to profit most from a favorable result.

What would that result mean for you? It could mean that a doctor might say, "Well, we finally got this straightened out, after many years of not knowing for sure. It's really clear that Brand X is the best, so I'm switching you to it. It works great for many of my other patients, so now I think it's time for you to move from your current brand to Brand X." We submit to you that Brand X may or may not be better for you. Here's why.

The research that yielded this result almost certainly did not find that every person tested did better with Brand X. That is not what happens in even the best research studies. What happens is that some people do better on Brand X, some on Brand Y, some on Brand Z. Some evidently do better on natural thyroid, and others may even do better on various combinations of natural and synthetic hormone medication.

Suppose the conclusion of the research study was that 67 percent of the people did best on Brand X. Okay, that's fairly compelling.

But how about the other 33 percent who did better on something else? How does your doctor know that you're not one of the 33 percent who would do better on something other than Brand X? You won't know until you try it for yourself.

Even if many studies confirm that Brand X is best for 67 percent of the population, that doesn't mean that it will ever be the best for you. This simple fact, which seems so obvious to us, is evidently lost on many of our colleagues. We are not talking about anecdotal evidence here. We are talking about what is true for one particular person on the planet—you.

Tell your doctor whether or not you feel good on the brand he or she has selected for you. If you're not doing well with your current brand of thyroid, ask to switch to a different brand. If you are on a generic product and are not doing as well as you would like, ask for one or more of the brand name medications. Realize that each "try" should be given at least five or six weeks before you draw any conclusion about its effectiveness, unless the trial of the new medication is making you feel terrible.

A significant number of people might not do well, no matter what brand or dose of thyroxine they take. The best improvement some people achieve with thyroxine alone is only 60 or 80 percent of their former sense of well-being.

This is still a significant improvement over how they might feel on no medicine at all. Suppose their doctor says, "Listen, this improvement is as good as we can do. This is what you have to expect with this illness: the medicine doesn't cure the condition, it just manages it. You must learn to live with it."

The patient can respond, "Wait a second. How do I know that this is as good as it can be? Thyroxine is only one of several kinds of thyroid hormones used to treat this condition. What if I could be at

90, or maybe even 95 percent improvement, with a different medication?" It may take time to refine your program until you are adequately improved.

The informed patient has a right to be included and considered in
all decisions. If your physician does not agree with something you
believe, the onus is on him or her to show you the research data and
allow you time to review and determine for yourself what you would
like to do. You have the right for your opinion to be respected.

Various Medical Options

Suppose you and your doctor decide to try a different medication.
What might it be? A different kind of synthetic thyroid hormone is
called Cytomel. This is synthetic T-3 thyroid hormone, and occasionally it works better for some people than the synthetic T-4. It is
pure fast-acting thyroid hormone, and—microgram for microgram—
is considered to be four times as strong as the slow acting thyroxine.

If you were on 100 micrograms of Synthroid, and not doing as
well as you'd like, you might want to see how life would be with a
switch to 25 micrograms of Cytomel.[1] As with all thyroid medications, you will need to try several doses in order to find the best level
for you.

Cytomel comes in tablets of 5, 25, and 50 microgram strength. It
is not currently used by itself as often as it was in the past. Because it
is active thyroid hormone, it is quick-acting. This results in some
people having a jagged response: their blood may contain high levels
of medication shortly after taking the pill, and lower levels later during the day. As a result, their level of symptom relief can fluctuate
widely.

For other people, Cytomel can be a little too stimulating for the heart. They might develop palpitations. For many, however, it can be exactly what is needed. It certainly avoids possible difficulties in converting T-4 into T-3. With Cytomel, there is no conversion problem at all, since it is active T-3 thyroid hormone in the first place. By taking the active component, you avoid having to convert it prior to benefiting from it.

If you find that you do not tolerate Cytomel, or that it is no more effective than thyroxine, then you have the option of Thyrolar. In fact, there used to be two similar medications: Thyrolar and Euthroid. Euthroid is no longer available, and Thyrolar is increasingly hard to find.

Thyrolar represents the intriguing therapeutic combination of synthetic T-3 and synthetic T-4. Sometimes this combination, which is similar to the combination of T-3 and T-4 circulating in the normal bloodstream, is more powerful than T-3 or T-4 alone. This combination therapy, although not yet endorsed by some doctors and pharmacists, seems to be very beneficial in certain patients.

The one big problem with Thyrolar is that, although it comes in three dosages, the ratio of T-3 to T-4 is a fixed combination, making it more difficult to do a good titration. A far better maneuver is to have two bottles of medicine, one bottle containing synthetic T-4, the other bottle containing synthetic T-3. Using two different medications, you can get a dual titration that might be more fine-tuned than anything that you've tried so far. You can then experience what 1 microgram per pound of T-4 feels like, combined with 5 or 10 total micrograms of Cytomel. This combination method allows for sensitive individuals to fine-tune their prescription to suit their individual needs.

Combining T-4 and T-3 is useful for people who have not been doing as well on either medication alone. In fact, it seems to have some very definite advantages, and should be tried if other maneuvers are not satisfactory.

Recently, research demonstrating the increased efficacy of the combination of T-3 and T-4 was published in the prestigious *New England Journal of Medicine*.[2] The research represented such a departure from the standard view that it was accompanied by an editorial opening the topic to further discussion.

This brings us to a very important point. We believe that any thyroid medicine you have tried with some success can be combined with any other thyroid medicine that you have tried with some success. The benefit of the combination may be much greater than the benefit of either medication alone. We certainly do not recommend this elaborate a maneuver for anyone who does not really need it. However, if you have tried repeatedly to find relief from the multiple symptoms of a well-diagnosed thyroid problem, we urge you to use whatever will give you maximal improvement.

Natural Thyroid

Suppose there is no combination of different synthetic thyroid medications that works really well for you. Would you consider trying animal thyroid (also called natural thyroid)?

Many patients prefer animal or natural thyroid to synthetic thyroid, even though it is not currently the standard in this country.[3] Years ago, all low thyroid patients in the United States were on it, because it was the only product available. Now, natural thyroid is used more commonly in various other countries, especially Western Europe. It is very popular among practitioners of alternative and complementary medicine in the United States. The Broda Barnes M.D. Research Foundation in Trumbull, Connecticut (see Resources), can supply you with information from the world medical literature to support Dr. Barnes's view that natural thyroid might even have advantages over any amount of synthetic.

Some people say this issue of synthetic versus natural thyroid is akin to the debate regarding the use of synthetic versus organic fertilizers in farming. Those familiar with this debate have heard how fertilizing a garden or field with just the three standard synthetic chemicals is not nearly as beneficial as growing plants organically with compost (which contains hundreds of different natural chemicals, not simply three synthetically derived ones). If you've ever eaten fruit or vegetables grown from a composted garden, as opposed to those from a synthetically fertilized garden, you may be convinced of the superiority of the former. It turns out that large farms can use the natural method as well, and the resulting food has been shown to be more nutritious.

Taking desiccated animal thyroid gland (natural thyroid) might also supply a person with useful intermediary substances such as T-1 and T-2 thyroid hormone, in addition to the final products called T-3 and T-4. Some patients seem to need the intermediary substances; others do not. It is up to you to ascertain if natural thyroid works better in your particular body.

The most common brand of natural thyroid is called Armour, though it is not the only brand. It has been in existence for many years, having been passed around from one drug company to another as a less lucrative medicine. Apparently, it does not make as much money as the synthetic brands, but it has been kept on the market because of the significant minority of people who do better with it.

Another brand of natural thyroid is Westhroid, which is perhaps more "organic" than Armour. By this we mean that the animals that were the source of thyroid were raised without being given hormones or antibiotics and were fed grain grown without herbicides, pesticides, or artificial fertilizer. You can have your pharmacy order this version of thyroid for you, if what they have available (usually Armour or a generic natural product) has not given you satisfactory results. Other brand-name natural thyroid medicines are also occasionally available.

Consider the case of Christine, who had been on Synthroid for five years without fully regaining her prediagnosis strength and stamina. Her doctor examined her test results carefully and was very open-minded regarding treatment options. When she tried more of the thyroxine, she had worse insomnia and developed a skin rash. She dropped back to a milder dose. Fortunately, she had a doctor who was astute enough to add some Cytomel. This gave her a slight improvement, but the Synthroid-Cytomel combination did not have her feeling nearly as energetic as she had felt before the onset of the hypothyroidism.

Christine asked her doctor for a trial of natural thyroid. He was not very hopeful but eventually agreed. The switch in her medication turned out to be very successful. After only two weeks on Armour thyroid, she felt better than she had felt during the five years she'd spent on synthetic thyroid. Even the last year of taking the Synthroid-Cytomel combination was not nearly as productive. Her benefit increased over the next several weeks. Eventually, she regained full functional capacity in body and mind. She said it felt like a miracle, and only wished that she had tried natural thyroid earlier.

Bolstered by Christine's outstanding success, we put our very next new patient needing medication onto Armour thyroid, rather than starting with a synthetic. Ironically, the Armour thyroid didn't work as well with this patient. In fact, it seemed to be only slightly better than no medicine at all. When she was switched from the natural to the synthetic thyroid, she felt terrific. Many others in our practice felt great on Armour from the very beginning.

Be an Actualized Patient

As you can see, thyroid sufferers are very idiosyncratic in their response to medication. It is important for you to experiment so as to discover the treatment that is just right for your particular biochemistry.

We can readily understand why many providers would not want to practice in this manner. It is extremely time consuming, requiring a vast wellspring of patience to monitor each patient's fluctuating progress. The process demands that the caregiver walk side by side with the patient, educating and supporting the person who is in the midst of this (sometimes) roller-coaster existence. The managed care environment does not allow practitioners to devote the careful attention that is called for to find just the right dose of just the right medicine(s) for each person.

In addition, the patients aren't usually acutely ill. Their condition is more of a longstanding, chronic condition that moves slowly. Some health care providers do not have patience for this mild situation.

It is also risky for the doctor to step out of the standard mold, and try something slightly different. Physicians are monitored and are expected to practice in accordance with a certain community standard. That means that if seven general practitioners in a given city never prescribe anything but synthetic thyroid, and the eighth GP sometimes uses synthetics and sometimes uses natural thyroid, that eighth doctor is not considered to be practicing in accordance with the standards of the community. The actual legal risk is minimal, yet it still discourages many doctors from innovation. We believe that the reverse should be true: that the other seven should be held accountable for not practicing up to the proper standard. Sadly, it is the eighth doctor who is legally at risk.

Caring for highly sensitive patients requires an ability to express empathy and concern, to share information, and to expose oneself to the subtle intricacies of the patient's life. We know from personal experience that we have to be taking good care of ourselves in order to sustain that level of interaction without burning out.

Doctors are also rightly concerned with how their actions are perceived by patients. The "feel your way" approach is not how physicians are taught to act in medical school. In fact, Richard recalls one of his medical professors advising young doctors never to say, "I don't know." They were told to say anything intelligent-sounding, rather than admit they didn't know something.

Doctors are trained to think that an omniscient demeanor is most reassuring to the patient. In some cases this is true, perhaps mostly with older patients, who have been indoctrinated to believe the doctor is infallible. We believe that our job is to educate and motivate, rather than dictate. The doctor should be open-minded, willing to try a variety of different medicines, and to help the patients decide which one is really working best for them.

We consider that part of our role as caregiver is to empower and honor the individuals who seek our knowledge, wisdom, and support in safeguarding their health. It is well documented that patients' beliefs play an integral role in healing. It is also well documented that an empowered patient does much better than one who simply follows orders (see one of the many fine books written by Yale oncology surgeon Bernie Siegel, M.D.).

People come to physicians from many families, cultures, backgrounds, and institutions, each of which influences their belief system. To be effective in working collaboratively, practitioners must take the time to understand and explore their patients' beliefs. Caregivers can save a great deal of time and energy by listening carefully in the initial interview so as to find common ground and define a meaningful framework for treatment. This is done with an open mind and heart.

We operate from a deeply held conviction that in the long run each person is his or her own best physician. Practitioners may have greater medical knowledge and technical expertise, but there is no one who knows more about what is best for this patient, on the deepest level, than the patient. He or she has traveled roads on the life journey that we have not. The health challenges he or she faces are a part of that journey, and practitioners are privileged to be able to grow and learn from the people they work with.

Our job is to inspire in our patients what we call the "will to be well." We cannot heal them; we can work alongside them for their own healing. And we can empower them with skills, tools, information, and support.

We strongly consider that what the patients believe to be good, or not good, for them is of utmost value in planning our approach. If patients have had negative experiences with certain medications, we respect their concerns and experiences. We encourage health care consumers to be sure to articulate feelings and beliefs about treatment. If your health care provider is not interested in hearing your feelings or beliefs, you may want to consider whether you are working with the right person.

Timing Is Everything

It is important when—and how—you take thyroid medicine. Taking it in the morning, a half hour before eating, often works best. You are certainly free to experiment, but absorption of medication is more complete if pills are taken on an empty stomach long before food, vitamins, or any other supplements.

Another aspect of timing relates to duration of therapy. How long might you expect to stay on your thyroid pills? Not all sufferers of simple low thyroid need to be on their medication forever. For some, it can be a temporary maneuver, lasting a few months to a few years. For others, it is definitely a lifelong recommendation.

Generally, severe autoimmune thyroiditis is treated forever. Milder versions might do well with a shorter duration of therapy. This is especially true if you include into your overall health program some of the nonprescription activities discussed later in this book. Always work with a good health care provider before discontinuing your thyroid hormone.

A Caution About Generic Medications

Regardless of whether there are differences in effectiveness among the three leading brand name thyroxines, it has been found that these brands work better than generic thyroid medications. This is true not only at our office but at other medical institutions as well. Generic thyroid is a bit less expensive but has often been less effective. There are certain generic drugs that seem to be just as effective as their brand-name counterparts, but in the thyroid arena, this does not appear to be the case. If you are on a managed care plan that insists on using generic drugs, and you are not doing as well as you would like with your thyroid, firmly request the brand name.

An unusual twist in the brand versus generic thyroid discussion is the issue of Levoxyl, mentioned earlier. Since this very good brand-name thyroxine is less expensive than other brands, it is sometimes used as a substitution for Synthroid or Levothroid. Because it is an excellent medication, it is always worth a try. In fact, many doctors and patients consider it their first choice.

What's Next?

If you have tried as many different doses, brands, or combinations as you think are appropriate and are still not doing as well as you would like, it's time to look further. It is possible that prescription thyroid hormone might only partially improve your sense of well-being. If it doesn't help you get where you want to go, it could be time to look for imbalances in other hormones.

Keep in mind that the endocrine system is a complex, exquisitely interconnected network, with each gland in communication with the others. If treatment with thyroid hormone alone is not sufficient for your needs, it is possible that other glandular challenges are complicating your situation. Accordingly, the next step will focus on reproductive glands, followed by a step on restoring the adrenals.

The Bottom Line

- There is no one "best medicine" for all low thyroid sufferers.
- Each person needs to ascertain, largely by trial and error, which medication works best in his or her system.
- Sometimes what works best is a combination of two different medications.
- Sometimes what works best now may not work as well later. Optimal dosing is an ongoing process.
- People with mild low thyroid may not need to take prescription medication forever, although many find it most beneficial to do so.

Reestablish Balance in Your Reproductive System

In all cases of organic deficiency—the body is borne like a burden; a hostile stranger—

—SIMONE DE BEAUVOIR, *The Second Sex*

This step is divided into two main sections. The first addresses female reproductive issues related to low thyroid, such as menstrual problems, fertility, menopause, and sexual enjoyment. The second deals with male issues, rarely discussed, yet also vitally important.

The Goddess in Distress

Most people would be surprised to discover the extent to which the thyroid is intimately related to a satisfying sex life. Moreover, the entire success or failure of your reproductive function depends on the proper working of this important gland in your neck.

Many women today—especially menopausal women—are echoing a common refrain: "There must be something wrong with my hormones." The problem is not simply that women are living longer and some need added estrogen in their later years. The reality is much more complex, and it frequently involves the thyroid gland.

Proper diagnosis and treatment of hypothyroidism could go a long way toward alleviating menstrual and sexual difficulties, but many people who could benefit from treatment are scared away because of the misconception (see step 5) that proper thyroid treatment will cause osteoporosis. It is our hope that this chapter will shed new light on the help that thyroid treatment can offer women who suffer from problems related to menstruation, fertility, or sexual enjoyment.

"What's Wrong with My Hormones?"

Just as low thyroid can cause poor function of the digestive system, or the musculoskeletal system, improper amounts of thyroid hormone can have a variety of deleterious effects on the reproductive system. Thyroid hormone is the gas pedal for the thousands of other chemical reactions in the body. It influences every organ and cell.

In fact, it is for this very reason that many people, especially women, are not properly diagnosed. Because the thyroid underlies so many diverse functions of the body, it is often completely ignored. How could such a terrible thing happen? A middle-aged woman might visit her doctor, complaining of heavy periods, muscle aches, stiff joints, severe dry skin, vaginal itching, headaches, difficulty with digestion, and inability to concentrate. She is very liable to be labeled as a "kook," or be told, "There, there, you're just going through menopause."

It is difficult for many medical professionals to believe that all these disparate symptoms could be traced to a singular treatable disease process. Doctors are trained to put a patient's multiple difficulties into one tidy, recognizable box in order to arrive at a logical explanation for the presenting complaints.

Managed care magnifies or worsens this dilemma, demanding that doctors pigeonhole the patient's diagnosis, assigning it a numerical code (e.g., 564.1 = irritable bowel syndrome). If the patient's symptoms do not nicely match the insurance company's description, the physician's dilemma is either to change the diagnosis to fit the problem, consider that the patient is somehow mentally unstable, or tell the truth, which could result in nonreimbursement (for the patient or physician).

While it might seem straightforward to a thyroid specialist to put all of these diverse symptoms into the category "245.2: autoimmune low thyroid," most primary care doctors are not sufficiently thyroid suspicious. Endocrine function in general is not adequately taught in medical school and is rarely in the forefront of internship and residency training. In addition, primary care providers are geared toward diagnosing life-threatening situations and do not devote as much attention to these "minor" irritating symptoms.

Many women have told us that their response to this unfortunate prevailing trend is to hold back disclosure of some of their symptoms related to periods or emotions, so as not to be dismissed as merely menopausal or depressed. For generations, given the patriarchal nature of the medical system, it was common practice for doctors not to put much stock in what their female patients told them. In fact, not many years ago, women were committed to mental institutions for voicing such a battery of complaints.

Libido Woes

Low levels of thyroid hormone affect women's sexual desire as well as the quality of sexual activity. Less thyroid hormone means less sex. Inadequate amounts of thyroid hormone translate into an improper balance of the essential female hormones. The result is less sexual interest, less sexual fantasy, less response to sexual stimulation, and less sexual excitement, in part related to the effect of low thyroid on the prerequisite brain chemicals. Moreover, the autonomic nervous system, responsible for engorgement and lubrication of sexual organs, functions less well when thyroid is low.

Hypothyroid women can even cease to ovulate and may experience severe vaginal dryness, making intercourse (when it does occur) painful. All too frequently, a woman with vaginal dryness is told, "Oh, your estrogen is too low. Here is the latest hormone replacement therapy" (HRT). Commonly, when thyroid is low, HRT will not help sufficiently. What this woman needs is to have her thyroid corrected. After that, she may not need estrogen at all.

Also killing sexual desire is the inner experience a woman has while hypothyroid. She is exhausted, feels depleted, is likely losing hair, gaining weight, and feeling quite bloated. Just ask that woman how sexy she feels! Over and above all this, low thyroid can, in itself, cause depression, hardly a fertile ground for a great sex life.

Some physicians believe that once the thyroid imbalance is corrected, these difficulties in sexual desire improve, eventually returning to normal. Others believe that the woman experiences a form of post-traumatic stress syndrome, with a certain interval of continuing depression, despite adequate thyroid and estrogen treatment.

We believe that women who do not experience full recovery

with thyroid medications alone would see the expected improvement with a more holistic program. This would include options we will discuss in later steps, such as vitamins and mineral supplementation, an exercise schedule, and stress reduction strategies, as well as adrenal supplementation and attention to the autoimmune issue.

Menstrual Miseries

Low thyroid function has been documented as associated with menstrual disorders for well over a hundred years. Everything from excessive blood flow and severe cramps to irregular cycles has been corrected, at least in some women, with the addition of thyroid hormone. The weaker a woman's thyroid function, the greater her menstrual blood loss and cyclical irregularity.

Although there are many other possible causes for menstrual difficulties (examples: fibroids, ovarian cysts, cervical polyps, endometriosis), in most women experiencing menstrual problems, there is no evidence of these organic disorders. What is found, if adequately suspected, is low thyroid, the treatment of which frequently relieves the problem. In fact, thyroid treatment has probably cured more menstrual disorders than all other medications combined.

Many women who have had hysterectomies because of abnormal bleeding might have been able to save their uterus if hypothyroidism had been diagnosed and treated. Once again, unless the often unreliable blood tests show a woman is low thyroid, she may be denied thyroid treatment. Relying simply on blood tests to diagnose a thyroid deficiency relegates many women unnecessarily to surgical treatment, either for D&C for dysfunctional bleeding, or a hysterectomy for intractable bleeding.

Missing the Diagnosis on Miscarriage

One of the most heartbreaking of all medical problems during a woman's childbearing years is the untimely loss of pregnancy. Some women have the devastating experience of one miscarriage after another. Miscarriages can be caused by inborn, environmental, or illness-related factors. Adequate amounts of thyroid hormone are essential for the maturation of the fetus and proper functioning of the uterus during pregnancy.

Low thyroid ranks high as one of the causes of miscarriage, especially when recurrent.[1] Even mild hypothyroidism can cause repeated miscarriage. In fact, a woman can have a light case of Hashimoto's thyroiditis that does not cause her thyroid hormone levels to be low, yet this may well be the cause of her miscarriage.[2]

In twenty-five years of medical practice, we have seen a number of these unfortunate situations be completely reversed with the simple—and long overdue—addition of thyroid hormone. One of our patients, Betty, had two miscarriages when she consulted us at the beginning of her third pregnancy. No cause for the prior miscarriages had been determined, despite an extensive workup by a very good OB-Gyn, specializing in high-risk pregnancy.

No one had previously suspected low thyroid function because her TSH was normal at 3.0 (typical range = 0.4–5.2). However, she had the classic symptoms of low thyroid: fatigue, low stamina, dry skin, and a sense of feeling chilly most of the time. Additional tests at our clinic revealed significant levels of antithyroid antibodies, and a Total T-3 thyroid hormone level of 72 (borderline low).

We started her on a very low dose of Armour thyroid hormone that was gradually and conservatively increased under close monitoring by both her obstetrician and us. Like many other women with a history of miscarriage and symptoms of low thyroid, she responded beautifully. Not only did she feel better during this pregnancy after starting thyroid medicine, but she carried the baby to term and had a normal birth.

We do not want to minimize the enormous difficulties that miscarriage presents to both patient and doctor. Nor do we, for a moment, believe that all miscarriage problems could be solved by taking thyroid medication. We fervently believe, however, that the case above is not a rare, isolated example.

Years ago, it was a common practice for obstetricians to administer thyroid hormone to women who were having miscarriages. Once treated, many of these women were able to deliver healthy, full-term babies. We believe this old practice should be reevaluated and tried more often. Better yet, women's thyroid levels should be more completely evaluated prior to pregnancy.

New Hope for Infertility

It is well documented that infertility has been increasing over the past few decades. One suspected cause of this statistical rise is related to the increase in the prevalence of untreated low thyroid. One researcher has reported that as many as one quarter of the women being treated at a well-known fertility clinic had borderline low thyroid.[3]

Yet, women suffering fertility problems are not tested for low thyroid as rigorously as this statistic would seem to mandate. Fertility clinics in the past commonly put many women on low dose thyroid replacement, regardless of test results. Although this might have appeared to be unwarranted medicalization of a patient, the outcome was generally favorable. These days, women who are just starting with fertility specialists are not routinely placed on thyroid. Neither are they tested for it in as thorough and detailed a manner as we would wish. This oversight has resulted in a great many women spending enormous amounts of time and money on multiple other drugs and procedures, often with unpleasant side effects and disappointing results.

Lorrie's experience is rather common. She underwent fertility evaluation and treatment not once, but at two separate times. Each was a two-year ordeal of multiple blood draws, hormone injections, and weeks of anxious waiting, all to no avail.

When she finally came to our office, it was not for fertility purposes but for a long overdue general checkup. Her menstrual history revealed long term irregularity, in addition to her inability to get pregnant. A detailed family history revealed one aunt and two cousins diagnosed with low thyroid. When asked if she had been tested for hypothyroidism, she said "Yes, and I was normal."

More extensive testing through our office confirmed normal blood levels of thyroid, but the results were now, and had been in the past, borderline low. We asked Lorrie if she would like to try thyroid hormone, to see if this would regularize her cycle and possibly support a pregnancy. She was hesitant because of her history of disappointments, but decided to try thyroid medication.

Once she was on thyroid hormone, her cycle normalized within two or three months. Her ovulatory temperature charts began to reflect a more normal monthly pattern, indicating she might now be fertile. Once she and her husband starting trying, she became pregnant in three months. Her pregnancy was uneventful, and nine months later she delivered a wonderful, sassy baby girl. (Lorrie later went on national television with her story, saying jokingly, "My GP got me pregnant.")

We are not the only practitioners who have discovered this simple relationship between thyroid and pregnancy. As noted by Dr. Ridha

Arem, a professor of endocrinology at Baylor Medical Center: "In the past four years, I have cared for five women with minimal hypothyroidism whose infertility problems were reversed within two to three months after they began thyroid hormone treatment. Prior to the thyroid problems being identified, all of them had suffered significant emotional and financial burdens [from infertility treatments] . . ."[4] Many case histories like this may be found in his book, *The Thyroid Solution* (see Further Reading).

We firmly believe that any man or woman dealing with fertility problems should have the thyroid connection evaluated thoroughly. In fact, even if the thyroid evaluation is "normal," they may want to consider a clinical trial of thyroid medication as Lorrie did and should work with a qualified, empathetic, and knowledgeable practitioner. The possible side effects of taking low-dose thyroid hormone are minimal. The possible benefits in this situation are enormous.

One very outspoken proponent of this course of action was Broda Barnes, M.D., the well-known thyroid specialist of the 1960s and 1970s. Throughout his many years of practice, Dr. Barnes had an unusually high success rate treating infertile couples. In fact, a good part of his success was due to his being able to recognize low thyroid in the husband as well as the wife.[5] We believe there may well be a link between the rise in infertility and the rise in untreated hypothyroidism over the past few decades. We urge anyone concerned about fertility to pay attention to what Dr. Barnes called "the unsuspected illness."

A Milder Menopause

Despite increased awareness in the medical community about the issues and interventions surrounding menopause, tremendous numbers of women still suffer from menopausal difficulties. They expend a great deal of time, money, and heartache on hormone replacement therapies. Frequently, neither the synthetic nor the natural hormones provides complete relief, because the underlying problem is undiagnosed low thyroid. By age fifty, one in every twelve women has a significant degree of hypothyroidism. By age sixty, it is one woman out of every six.[6]

This runaway thyroid epidemic seems to be striking menopausal women harder than any other group of patients. Fortunately, much can be done to help them. The standard maneuver by gynecologists is to provide a handful of estrogen samples to perimenopausal patients. We have heard too many stories of women in their late forties and early fifties who were given these hormones without any blood testing at all.

The compliant patient will follow the doctor's advice. But in cases where women have been put on estrogen, and the symptoms of hot flashes, insomnia, irritability, palpitations, and "fuzzy thinking" are still quite annoying, the addition of thyroid hormone can be a godsend. For symptomatic menopausal women not wanting or benefiting from estrogen, we advocate thyroid blood testing first, perhaps followed by a clinical trial of thyroid hormone, even if their blood tests are in the normal range.

Frequently the underlying hypothyroidism is such a controlling factor that simply correcting it returns the whole system to fairly normal functioning. Menopause continues, but it is a more mild, gradual, and comfortable process. If your thyroid is low, your hot flashes will be much more pronounced, much more frequent, and more disconcerting. This is because thyroid is your energy throttle, your gas pedal. You need energy to go through the change gracefully.

How much energy people have, how well they get up in the morning, how well they sleep, and how much stamina they have for the day is directly related to their levels of thyroid hormone. When your level is too low, you don't have the energy to cope adequately with anything, much less the additional stress and emotional lability associated with the menopausal years.

Consider the case of Sarah, a fifty-one-year-old schoolteacher. Both she and her mother started menopause at what would be considered an early age of forty-six. Sarah knew that her mother had low thyroid, as well as severe menopause problems. Neither the mother, nor Sarah, nor their doctors connected these two situations. When Sarah herself began to have the same severe menopause problems as her mother, she accepted it as her genetic predisposition. She was sometimes so hot and sweaty during a school day that she would need to keep a change of clothes in the teachers' lounge. Needless to say, the kids got on her nerves easily, and she was not enjoying her previously satisfying job.

Faced with these difficulties, Sarah did what her mother had not done: she began taking Premarin and Provera immediately. The hoped-for relief, however, was only minimal, even when the gynecologist increased her dosage. Fortunately, she was referred to our office by her school principal, who was our patient. Sarah's previously normal TSH was now, with advancing menopause, 6.2, clearly in the abnormal range. It indicated that her thyroid hormone levels were not keeping up with the extra demands of her changing metabolism.

Once on thyroid medication, she began to feel like her old self in a matter of weeks. Her menopause symptoms faded into the background, and her life became more balanced and enjoyable. Best of all, she no longer needed the Premarin and Provera to maintain this more graceful version of menopause. Thyroid hormone alone resolved the problems.

Other menopausal symptoms are equally amenable to treatment

with thyroid hormone alone. Atrophic vaginitis, or thinning of the vaginal wall as the result of falling estrogen levels, can lead to itching, discharge, and painful intercourse. All of these symptoms are much more severe when your thyroid is low. Women who have had unremitting vaginal dryness that was unresolved with vaginal creams or estrogen pills are often found to be low thyroid, if checked carefully. In addition to getting an important part of their intimate life back, once treated with thyroid medicine, these women are pleased to find that their problems with dry hair, dry skin, and cracking nails are often resolved as well.

An interesting ally of thyroid medication in some of these instances is natural progesterone. According to John Lee, M.D., in his book *What Your Doctor May Not Tell You About Menopause,* natural progesterone cream can augment the benefits of thyroid replacement therapy. This is, of course, in addition to its beneficial effects on menopause symptoms directly. Many women who have used thyroid hormone alone or progesterone cream alone may find their residual menopause difficulties disappear entirely when the two are used together. Just remember, too much estrogen opposes thyroid function, while natural progesterone is supportive of it.

Another medical authority who thinks that low thyroid is a crucial but often overlooked menopause issue is Christiane Northrup, M.D. In her wonderful book, *Women's Bodies, Women's Wisdom,* she makes a strong case for women who are having any kind of persistent menopause difficulty to be tested (and perhaps retested) for hidden low thyroid.

We don't intend to belittle the persistent difficulty that some women have at this time in their life. Not everyone will be helped as quickly or as completely as was Sarah. The dance of the hormones is very complex, so the idea that you can take just one hormone, or even two, and experience total relief is not always borne out successfully. You need to look at the whole picture. That's what we mean by holistic health.

Try to take into account all of your hormones, not just one of them. In fact, you can use this multifactored approach to assess all aspects of your life when trying to solve a thorny problem. If you are dissatisfied with your relationship or your job, these could be crucial aspects of your return to a less symptomatic menopause. Many women find that more than medical intervention is needed. Some find that quiet time away from their life stressors works wonders. Another reason to look beyond simple estrogen replacement is the fact that estrogen is not always a friendly and helpful substance. Contrary to what the pharmaceutical industry and your doctors may be telling you, estrogen's benefits have been overrated and its risks minimized.

There is the grave concern of the relationship between estrogen replacement and cancer in women. While estrogen has long been touted as a solution to the increased risk of heart disease in menopausal women, recent evidence suggests that this benefit has been much overplayed.

Thyroid hormone, in contrast, has never been causally linked to female cancers. Nor does it cause breast discomforts or life-threatening blood clots. It is safe and inexpensive. We urge you to consider trying thyroid hormone prior to starting estrogen therapy, if you have any suspicion at all of low thyroid, particularly if your family or personal medical history indicates that you have risk factors that contraindicate estrogen therapy.

Many women are disturbed to discover, besides the possible deleterious side effects, that Premarin is made from pregnant mares' urine. These horses are kept in a tight stall with an indwelling catheter to catch all of the urine. This lack of exercise and dignity can continue for the duration of the mare's life. Once the mare drops her foal, which is often slaughtered, she is soon reimpregnated and put back into the tight stall with the indwelling catheter. This unsavory practice is not reserved for a few odd horses here and there. One particular company's operation involved nearly a hundred thousand animals. Premarin is one of the top-selling drugs in this country.

Men's Issues: The Wounded Warrior

Why should men be interested in low thyroid, when it is considered to be a woman's illness? First of all, low thyroid is not entirely a woman's illness. Men do get diagnosed with the condition, though much less frequently than women. It can affect them in similar ways, and occasionally may be just as severe.

The Odd Couple

Frequently, low-thyroid women have low-thyroid husbands, and high-thyroid women have high-thyroid spouses. Odd as this may be, a famous example is George and Barbara Bush, who were both hyperthyroid. Even their dog was hyperthyroid! All three of them had Graves' disease, a form of hyperthyroidism (high thyroid).

For reasons that are not entirely clear, a man who is married to an overtly low-thyroid woman often seems to have symptoms of borderline low thyroid himself. This rather odd situation seems unlikely for an illness that is clearly not contagious. Many men in these relationships are never diagnosed. Nevertheless, it is our belief that it happens far too often to be considered a coincidence.

As far as we can ascertain, people tend to select partners with similar energy levels. It would be hard for a mildly low-thyroid person to sustain a relationship with a high-thyroid person. The hyperthyroid person would want to get up early, go do some work, go to the zoo, take in a show, then have dinner, go to a late movie, meet some friends after that for drinks and might embark on a project later, once home. The hypothyroid person might prefer to get up late, amble out to get the paper, spend an hour over breakfast and coffee, and go back to bed with a magazine. Is this a marriage that could work?

What about men who do not have low thyroid themselves but are with someone who does? For optimal satisfaction in their relationship, it would be helpful for them to understand what their partner is up against. A man in this situation must realize that he cannot take everything his partner says so personally. Her hypothyroidism may actually cause her to have altered perceptions about herself and others, causing her to be periodically more critical, irritable, and less patient. She is fatigued, sometimes depressed, generally moody, and needs additional help to get things done. When she becomes very tired, she can feel that her brain isn't functioning well, causing her to make less than wonderful decisions at times. A man can handle these changes more effectively if he understands the complexity of her metabolic slowdown.

Intimate Relations with Hypothyroid Women

Low-thyroid women often have a lowered sex drive, sometimes lower self-esteem, lower energy, and lower stamina for sex. Frequently they have ceased having sexual fantasies or sexual feelings. They may take longer to be aroused and lubricate. Or, they may feel too exhausted to be interested. Many women plagued by hypothyroid symptoms are more interested in getting to sleep than in having sex with their man. All is not lost, however, especially if the man knows what to do in such a situation.

Many low-thyroid women find their sexual response is not gone, just buried. A patient, understanding partner can unearth some of this libido for their mutual benefit. Just cuddling and talking can help her to feel more close and cared for. She may be bombarded with emotions, some related to her man, others related to her sense of self, body image, or low self-esteem.

She may need to share these in a safe atmosphere before love-making can be initiated. Because of the many aches and pains she experiences much of the time, a few minutes of loving massage can help her relax her muscles. To feel comfortable with her body may be the best insurance for sex to remain an option. In this instance, massage oil from a health food store (without synthetic chemicals) can serve a variety of purposes, including lubrication of the skin and other dry tissues. This makes the massage and foreplay more enjoyable.

Some women with low thyroid find that they have more energy for sex in the morning before work starts, rather than after a full, exhausting day. Some find they are revived by light exercise in the evening, followed by a bath or hot tub. Many would rather go straight home after dinner, rather than stay out for a movie or socializing. They can be embarrassed by their constant exhaustion, and an earlier bedtime might allow for more relaxation and more sex.

Decreased Male Desire and Impotence: Could It Also Be Thyroid?
Nothing decreases sexual performance more than drugs, alcohol, and depression. Not even the peripheral vascular challenge of diabetes is

such an affront to the male capacity. Frequently, however, the substance abuse and depressed feelings are a result of a sluggish metabolism. Let us explain.

Men with low thyroid do not generally feel the same degree of dramatic exhaustion, chilliness, and dry skin as women. Instead, they often experience a more general slowdown that they decline to talk about, or even acknowledge. To keep up their former level of activity, they may seek the use of substances to help them get through the day. Unfortunately, however, this choice usually backfires.

Low thyroid hormone has direct effects on a man's sexual performance and health. A man may experience an inability to achieve erection, inability to sustain an erection, inability to ejaculate, or have a low sperm count. An even greater sexual downer is the low libido/low performance due to chronic depression. As we explained in Step 2, low thyroid can either be a direct cause of depression, or can worsen an existing depression from other causes.

Good-bye, Viagra!

Men are often too proud to admit or even realize that they are depressed. Even if they do suspect the diagnosis, many view asking for help as a sign of weakness. If you men reading this are suffering from any of the symptoms outlined above, take heart and realize that you are not alone. Researchers believe that many men suffer with these problems in silence.

Worldwide, a decline in sperm count levels has been identified, as well as an even more disconcerting increase in prostate cancer. Some physicians believe that the decrease in male fertility is related to the widespread increase in low thyroid. In addition, the uncomfortable escalation of male violence is attributed, by some, to aberrant testosterone metabolism, another hormone affected by thyroid function.

There is good news, however. Taking thyroid hormone is simple, safe, and inexpensive. It sometimes works even better for men than it does for women. Many of the men in our clinic had a smoother course of treatment and an easier time finding their optimal dose than the women did.

Considering the high cost of Viagra and other male potency boosters, the thyroid alternative is quite attractive. It may also be the most efficient way to fix the problems.

For example, suppose a red dashboard warning light comes on while you are driving. You may pull over and read your manual, or pull into a gas station for help. A less intelligent option might be to ignore it. An even less intelligent choice would be to say, "I don't like that red light. I'll cut the wire, so I won't have to keep looking at it." Impotence may well be a red dashboard light. Taking Viagra might be like ignoring the cause of the situation and continuing to drive. Taking stimulants and pep pills may be like cutting the wire, diminishing your connection with your body's vital natural energy source.

The Link Between Thyroid and Testosterone

It is quite possible that many male dysfunctions are related to low thyroid's pervasive effect on other organs. If your thyroid is low, you may have a low testosterone level as a result. What real man would stand for that? Taking thyroid hormone could therefore improve not just your low thyroid symptoms but also your low testosterone symptoms. However, there is a wrinkle in this scenario. Some men have a type of low thyroid that is not resolved by adding thyroid hormone alone. Instead, they never feel quite up to par, even if their hypothyroidism has been accurately diagnosed and well treated by competent physicians. What is missing for these particular men is the necessary complement of testosterone as a chemical enabler, allowing the thyroid hormone to do its fullest job.

Alberto was forty-six years old when he first came to see us. He had been diagnosed and treated at the Stanford Medical Center for hypothyroidism, which also ran in his family. He had experienced no sexual difficulties before, during, or after this treatment. Sexual response was not his problem.

Instead, he was tired and achy all over. His fatigue worsened when he tried to exercise, which in the past he had enjoyed tremendously. No amount of experimenting with different amounts, brands, and combinations of thyroid hormone gave him full relief. He just couldn't recapture the level of health he had felt before the onset of his hypothyroidism at age forty.

We decided to do a testosterone level assay on Alberto. This is a simple blood test that is best run by the lab as two separate determinations: total testosterone and free testosterone. The total testosterone measures the concentration of this hormone in the bloodstream. The free testosterone level (also called the free fraction) measures the amount of testosterone that is not bound tightly to bloodstream carrier proteins but is instead free to enter the cells immediately.

Alberto's total and free fractions both revealed a number at the lowest end of the normal range. *Pobrecito!* We recommended the addition of modest amounts of testosterone to his medical regimen. It worked beautifully. His full former self reemerged, much to his delight. He returned to daily exercise, now no longer tiring.

This example illustrates the importance of testosterone, and perhaps other hormones, for a man who is low thyroid. The glandular network is an interactive, delicate series of connections, all of which must be balanced for optimal health.

We have treated many men with Alberto's problem, with equally good results. We wonder just how many others might be out there, suffering needlessly, reluctant to have their problem checked carefully.

Male Menopause: Are We Kidding?

The answer is no. As some people have long suspected, men also have their own version of change of life. This is not the same as the psychological midlife crisis you may have heard or read about, although it may include it. We are referring to an actual physiological change that occurs in men. We believe that this syndrome, which takes many forms, occurs earlier and is more severe in the presence of a sluggish thyroid function.

The male menopause syndrome includes the following symptoms: taking longer to recover from illness, decreased exercise endurance, weight gain, decreased memory, thinning of hair, changes in sexual appetite. Many of these symptoms occur because levels of hormones and neuropeptides are diminishing at this stage of life, though not as dramatically as with women. Medical conditions can include enlarged prostate, increased body fat, and decreased muscle tone. In severe cases, a very few men respond to these changes with depression, and even suicide.

What can be done? First of all, increased awareness of the issue can lead to increased numbers of men getting tested for their thyroid and testosterone levels. Secondly, deficiencies in these hormones can then be easily and safely treated.

Finally, men and women alike can view daily challenges as a part of a larger process, one which fine-tunes and adjusts one's awareness of how to live a life of quality. In turn, this process can lead to both sexes finding their most powerful and creative selves.

The complex glandular dance initially described in this step will be further explored in our next step on the adrenal-thyroid connection. For now, please consider the self-assessment below. It offers both women and men the opportunity to determine if you need rebalancing of your sex hormones to achieve full benefit from your thyroid recovery program.

A Self-Assessment

For Women—in spite of good thyroid treatment, do you still have:

1. Breast swelling, tenderness, fibrocysts?
2. Hard-to-treat menopausal symptoms?
3. Weight gain for no obvious reason?
4. Acne that appears at specific times during your menstrual cycle?
5. Severe cramping at ovulation?
6. Increased urinary tract or vaginal infections?
7. Heavy/irregular periods?
8. Severe PMS?
9. Dark circles under the eyes?
10. Obvious water retention?
11. Joint and muscle pain?
12. History of fibroids, endometriosis, hysterectomy, or polycystic ovary disease?
13. History of miscarriage or infertility?
14. Inability to concentrate?
15. Poor sleep at night/fatigue during day?

If you marked four or more of these symptoms, your thyroid program may be further improved by additional balancing of your reproductive system. You may want to secure the assistance of an interested, qualified practitioner to guide you.

For Men—in spite of good thyroid treatment, do you still have:

1. Impotence or low sperm count?
2. Easy bruising?
3. Depression or significant memory loss?
4. Fatigue or sleepiness during the day for no obvious reason?
5. Desire to take something to boost your energy in the morning, and something to wind down at night?
6. Abnormal blood pressure?
7. Decreased stamina for sports or other physical activity?
8. A noticeable decrease in muscle tone or mass?
9. High cholesterol levels?
10. Loss of hair in places other than the head?
11. Longer recovery time from injury/illness?
12. Increased urinary frequency without significant prostate abnormality.

If you marked four or more of these symptoms, your thyroid program may be further improved by additional balancing of your reproductive system. You may want to secure the assistance of an interested, qualified practitioner.

The Bottom Line

- Proper diagnosis and treatment of low thyroid can generally improve the health of reproductive organs and sexual function.
- Specific problems with menstruation, libido, fertility, and miscarriage are frequently thyroid-related, and can often be effectively treated with thyroid hormone.
- Menopause, in particular, is one crucial area where low thyroid is commonly overlooked.
- Rebalancing female and male hormonal systems can frequently improve one's overall thyroid recovery program (for most women, this means less or no estrogen, and more natural progesterone).
- Male menopause, impotence, and prostate problems, can be dramatically eased with the proper combination of thyroid and male hormone balance.

Determine If Low Adrenal Should Also Be Treated

The thyroid is often affected during stress. Its hormones are among the most potent accelerators of chemical reactions in the body.

—HANS SELYE, M.D., *The Stress of Life*

By this point, you may have a definite sense that low thyroid is the cause of your bothersome symptoms. You may also now understand how low thyroid may have affected your other medical problems. It may even be that your practitioner considers the situation an open-and-shut case of low thyroid. If you have been prescribed the proper amounts of thyroid hormone—perhaps with additional substances to balance your reproductive system—and all is working well, you do not need attention to your adrenal glands.

If, on the other hand, you are not doing as well as you'd like, and especially if your symptoms have been somewhat atypical all along, then other factors need to be considered. One of the most important additional factors to take into account is your adrenal hormone level.

We will start with a simple explanation of adrenal gland location and function, and then explain why all of this is so important to your thyroid balance.

Why Focus on Adrenal Function?

Your adrenal glands are two pyramid-shaped pieces of tissue situated right above each kidney. Their job is to produce and release, when appropriate, certain regulatory hormones and chemical messengers. Adrenaline is manufactured in the interior of the adrenal gland, in an area called the adrenal medulla. The adrenal medulla is stimulated directly by nerves from the sympathetic portion of the autonomic nervous system, which regulates the "fight or flight" response.

The human body is able to respond immediately to threatening situations by generating a tremendous amount of energy in a hurry, enabling the person to run away quickly (flight), or face the threat (fight) with a massive influx of chemical support. These chemicals increase blood pressure, heart rate, and blood flow to muscles, while mobilizing sugar to burn. Nerve impulses from the brain cause the release of adrenaline from the adrenal gland, which helps you react appropriately in immediate short-term stress situations.

Cortisol, another chemical from the adrenal gland, is made in the exterior portion of the gland, called the adrenal cortex. Cortisol, commonly called hydrocortisone, is one of the most abundant—and one of the most important—of many adrenal cortex hormones. Cortisol helps you handle longer-term stress situations.

In addition to helping you handle stress, these two primary adrenal hormones, adrenaline and cortisol, along with others similarly produced, help control body fluid balance, blood pressure, blood sugar, and other central metabolic functions.

The adrenal cortex participates in an intricate hormone-feedback system, similar to that of the thyroid. It begins with the hypothalamus portion of the brain secreting a hormone called CRH (corticotropin releasing hormone). CRH travels to the adjacent pituitary, where it causes that gland to secrete corticotropin, called ACTH (adrenocorticotropic hormone).

ACTH then travels to the adrenal glands above the kidneys, where it stimulates secretion of cortisol and cortisol-related hormones. The amount of these hormones in the bloodstream ultimately controls, by a brain sensory mechanism, the amount of CRH released by the hypothalamus. In other words, when cortisone is low, CRH is released, triggering the entire cycle anew, and bringing the blood levels of cortisol back up to normal.

The Thyroid-Adrenal Connection

A major connection exists between low thyroid and low adrenal. Low adrenal, also called adrenal insufficiency, can actually cause someone's thyroid problem to be much worse than it would be otherwise.

Correction of low adrenal is similar to correction of low thyroid. You merely take a pill that contains some of the hormone you are lacking. The purpose of this chapter is to assure you that doing so, when appropriate, is not only safe and effective but can change your life for the better.

Cortisol is in the category of medicines called steroids, a class of body substances built upon the structure of the common cholesterol molecule. Both health practitioners and the lay public have great concern about the safety of taking oral steroids. We would like to address this issue directly by making a distinction between high-dose steroid therapy and low-dose adrenal supplementation.

What we are talking about in this book is the use of very small amounts of natural adrenal hormone (hydrocortisone) to bring slightly low adrenal function up to its proper normal daily range. This is in stark contrast to the high doses of powerful synthetic adrenal hormones commonly used to treat other health problems or to assist in building muscles.

Crucial Reasons for Knowing Your Adrenal Levels

Adrenal insufficiency symptoms include: weakness, lack of libido, allergies, dark circles under the eyes, muscle and joint pain, dizziness, low blood pressure, low blood sugar, food and salt cravings, poor sleep, dry skin, cystic breasts, lines of dark pigment in nails, difficulty recuperating from stresses such as colds or jet lag, no stamina for confrontation, tendency to startle easily, lowered immune function, anxiety, depression, and premature aging. Some of these symptoms are similar to those of low thyroid.

If low-thyroid people with these symptoms are put on thyroid hormone alone, they sometimes respond negatively. They may have coexistent but hidden low adrenal. If they take thyroid hormone by itself, the resultant increased metabolism may accelerate the low adrenal problem. The proper approach in this case is to treat the patient with thyroid and adrenal support simultaneously.

Adrenal insufficiency, especially when unmasked by the addition of thyroid hormone, is unpleasant and uncomfortable. To compound the problem, the doctor and patient then may wrongly assume that thyroid replacement has been a mistake. A tremendous opportunity for better health has now been missed.

While uncomfortable, this dilemma can become a diagnostic tool. The doctor could then gradually add thyroid and adrenal hormone together, with the patient eventually taking optimal levels of both. This careful attention and delicate calibration are demanding on the practitioner and patient. Nevertheless, we have seen patient after patient dramatically improve with such dedication.

Also, interactions among your hormones are sometimes as important as the direct action of the hormone itself. Some adrenal hormones assist in the conversion of T-4 to T-3 and perhaps assist in the final effect of T-3 on the tissues. Some scientists believe that even the entrance of thyroid hormone into our cells is under the influence of adrenal hormones. Thus, if your adrenal level is low enough, you might do well to take both adrenal and thyroid hormone together.

When Is Stress Useful to You?

As we've mentioned, the "fight or flight" response, controlled by adrenal hormones, is our adaptive and protective mechanism that converts energy into an immediate and effective response for overcoming danger. In seconds, you can shift biochemically into high gear, using adrenaline and related hormones to raise your blood pressure or summon the necessary muscular response needed to fight or flee danger.

In ages past, this mechanism was crucial for preservation of life and limb, as well as for securing food. Life in those primitive days was simpler than it is now. When an emergency situation occurred, it was met and dealt with immediately. Early men and women could then return to regular daily activity. The excess outpouring of adrenaline and cortisone was a sporadic, intermittent activity with plenty of recovery time in between.

Stress Versus Distress

Compared to ages past, life is dramatically more complicated now. People spend days, weeks and months in chronic, ongoing tension and anxiety. These mental states result in a physiology that has become downright illness provoking. Chronic stress and exhaustion are our reward for keeping up the pace in a complex society. In the 1950s, the famous researcher Hans Selye renamed this long-term fight or flight response "the general adaptation syndrome." He then went on to delineate much of our current knowledge about adrenal responses.

Selye divided the physiology of fight or flight into three phases. In the first phase, adaptation, a person intermittently secretes slightly higher levels of the fight or flight hormones in response to a slightly higher level of stress.

The second phase, called alarm, begins when the stress is constant enough, or great enough, to cause sustained excessive levels of certain adrenal hormones. This can be the very earliest glimmer of what later can become stress-induced illness.

The third phase is called exhaustion, wherein the body's ability to cope with the stress is now depleted. At this point, adrenal hormones plummet from excessively high to excessively low. It is this latter phase of adrenal exhaustion that sometimes accompanies or is confused with low thyroid.[1]

Where do low thyroid and adrenal stress intersect? If you find yourself in the alarm phase of adrenal stress (high levels of ACTH and high levels of cortisol), one result might be altered conversion of T-4 into T-3, or thyronine. Thus, your adrenal situation might profoundly affect the availability of biologically active thyroid hormone.

Research shows that even success and positive change can result in the stress response described above. In other words, even activities that you perceive as enjoyable, such as working hard on an exciting project, or striving for and receiving a promotion, can be perceived by the body as stress. This positive stress, called "eustress," can accumulate and affect bodily responses in the same way as its negative counterpart, "distress." In addition, some of the activities that are encouraged to help relieve this situation might actually make it worse.

Different Strokes for Different Folks

Sarah and Cathy were sisters. Both were on low-dose thyroid medication, and both had what appeared to be adrenal exhaustion from recent increased stress. Sarah, at age twenty-seven, was involved in an exciting but very demanding career. Unmarried and dating, she was busy day in and day out, morning, noon, and night, with enjoyable, challenging activity. But her pace suddenly became overwhelming when her company insisted that she transfer to another city and take on the managerial role for an entire department. Her promotion was welcome, but the extra stress of it was enormous.

She started to have difficulty coping with the inevitable challenges of moving her household: unpacking, searching for items that should have been in one place but instead were in another. At work, she had to deal with employees who were fearful of change and of losing their jobs because of the company's transition. Her normal easy-going disposition became combative, with hair-trigger eruptions. She had trouble going to sleep and would frequently wake up with a headache that interfered with her ability to concentrate most of the morning. She was clearly the victim of her adrenaline responses.

We suspect that she might have been in the adaptive phase before the move, burning the candle at both ends for years. As a high-energy person, perhaps she was still able to handle things successfully by running on higher than normal levels of adrenaline and cortisone. After the move, however, she became overwhelmed by the additional output of adrenal hormones, resulting in a maladaptive alarm phase that made her sick.

Her treatment, as recommended by a thoughtful practitioner, was to begin an exercise program. She was told this would help burn off the excess adrenaline and enable her to be more calm and cool under fire. The advice worked very well, and she returned to a more comfortable adrenal hormone level.

Contrast Sarah's experience with what happened to her sister. Cathy, at age thirty, had two young children. She was very involved in nurturing them and with their schooling, often volunteering on several committees. When her elderly mother sustained a stroke and had to move to a nursing home, things changed. Cathy's previous adaptation to the stresses of parenting had included the benefit of help from the elderly mother. Losing this support pushed her into stage two, alarm, and then into exhaustion. There was just too much to do and too many emotional ups and downs, with the added burden of visiting the nursing home. Cathy's exhaustion went on for many months, eventually leading to symptoms of skin rash, joint pains, and digestive difficulties.

On the advice of her sister, who had done so well improving her symptoms with an exercise program, Cathy signed up for one-on-one training at a local gym. The results were a disaster. Every one of her symptoms became exaggerated with the increase in exercise. She felt terrible most of the time. She did not understand why the same treatment that had been so helpful to her sister was so destructive to her. Thinking that she was just out of shape, she persisted, and her misery worsened.

The reason became apparent when Cathy came to our clinic for help. She was not in the alarm phase of adrenal depletion, needing to burn off excess adrenaline. Rather, she was in the exhaustion phase, and instead needed adrenal support and supplementation.

As you can see, the best advice for a person in adrenal exhaustion is not to exhaust the system further, depleting hormones that are already low. Instead, the best intervention is to restore the body chemicals that are deficient.

Mastering Stress and Creating Empowerment

The story of Sarah and Cathy illustrates the value of proper adrenal balance to your overall thyroid program. Our holistic perspective gives us a deep sense of the importance of these delicate interconnections, not only on the physical level, but on the level of emotions, thinking, and even on that difficult-to-describe aspect of our lives, the spiritual realm.

For many years, a dedicated scientist, Albert Bandura, Ph.D., has been quietly researching a topic called "empowerment" in the ivory towers of Stanford University Psychology Department. While his research is quite complex, the findings are amazingly relevant to our topic (see Further Reading) in that they address these holistic issues.

He began by educating spider-phobic women about spiders, so that eventually they were able to react less irrationally and physically handle them. How does this relate to you? First, it is important to remember that "stress" is not the same for every person. Stress is dependent upon our perceptions of how difficult a task is. Bandura found that three important things help us understand how we can make better decisions about our lives and reduce our stress.

Bandura measured the women's levels of catecholamines—adrenaline and the related blood chemicals involved in facing scary tasks—before, during, and after they were given information and support to overcome their fears. He found that the women's highest catecholamine levels occurred when they thought they couldn't do something but had to face it anyway. This is a common situation for many of us, especially those of us who are low thyroid and thus much more sensitive to our catecholamine levels than the average person.

Secondly, Bandura found that when people felt they couldn't do something and made the decision to refuse to try, their catecholamine levels dropped significantly. In other words, making the decision not to face the situation was empowering for them. Once they made a decision either to face a scary task or not to face it, their levels dropped significantly. The most stressful part was trying to figure out what to do.

Most powerful, however, was Bandura's third finding. He assessed women who felt unequal to facing a certain task and then provided what he called "mastery modeling," or having masters, or experts, demonstrate how to do something that might initially appear daunting. Gradually the women were desensitized to the scary task, becoming informed and practiced in dealing with the situation. These women had the lowest catecholamine levels of all.

Bandura later went on to study women during staged physical attacks by a specially trained "assailant." He found that when these women were provided with the skills, tools, information, and support to make healthier lifestyle choices, they no longer lived in fear or had continuously high levels of catecholamines. Bandura then took his inquiries even further, exploring the long-term benefits of this type of training. His findings are meaningful to us in this discussion of catecholamine balance. When women received mastery modeling in self-defense skills, they were no longer intimidated by situations that previously were terrifying.

Those who had been raped or assaulted and who had limited their lives as a result began to move out into a more expanded life. They were no longer afraid to go out at night, or to be in situations similar to those when they experienced the assault. This did not mean that they put themselves in harm's way. They knew they had skills to deal with these situations, but they also demonstrated greater powers of discernment. They were more acutely aware of which situations to avoid. In addition to facing stressful situations more easily, they also found that positive changes occurred in other areas of their lives. Having eliminated their phobic responses, they were able to secure better jobs, more pay, healthier relationships, and in general felt more powerful, and more productive in their lives.

Empowerment is about having the skills, tools, information, and support with which to make healthy changes. The purpose of this book is to empower you, the reader, to take action on your own behalf, and to have the knowledge and support to be effective as your own advocate for the best possible health care. This information is intended to reduce your stress level, increase your awareness of your situation, and teach you to communicate with your provider. To adequately address this thyroid issue, and the further complication of a possible thyroid-adrenal connection, it is essential that you not be under excessive stress while trying to address your stress levels!

Moreover, stress is ultimately the battle to remain normal in the face of any noxious agent. We want you to use this information about stress to better protect yourself from the many noxious agents now threatening your thyroid function (see Step 9).

How to Determine If You Are Low Adrenal

It would be wonderful to have a simple, reliable method of assessing a person's adrenal function. Many tests are available but none is widely used. One reason is that most medical doctors consider that the adrenal system is always functioning smoothly, except in two very severe and rare circumstances. One is caused by overproduction of cortisol called Cushing's Syndrome. Underproduction of cortisol is called Addison's Disease. When it is clear to a physician that you do not have either Cushing's or Addison's, the topic of adrenal metabolism all too often is shoved aside.

As you can see from the earlier discussion, normal adrenal metabolism is essential to good health, and problems can arise even when you do not have either of these two rare illnesses. The truth may well be that there is a continuum between these two extremes. Problems may occur at various points along this spectrum of adrenal dysfunction, rather than as rare illnesses that occur only at either extreme.[2]

Why Aren't Adrenal Tests Ordered More Often?
Another reason doctors may not be sufficiently involved in this topic is that adrenal tests are even more challenging to interpret than thyroid tests. The biochemistry is extremely complex and, until recently, the testing technology had not been widely useful except to diagnose Cushing's and Addison's. Now the measurements are more sophisticated. Current technology can be divided into roughly two camps:

conventional medical evaluation; and the more recently developed alternative adrenal tests.

What Are the Standard Options?

The conventional medical evaluation for adrenal function includes measurements of ACTH (adrenocorticotropic hormone) from the pituitary, as well as cortisol (hydrocortisone) from the adrenal glands themselves. Both of these are simple blood tests.

In addition, doctors will sometimes obtain a 24-hour urine sample for cortisol and related cortex hormones. Patients collect urine in the same large container every time they empty their bladder for an entire twenty-four-hour period. One drawback with this measurement is that it is not illustrative of variations within the twenty-four-hour period, because the whole day's worth of urine is mixed together in one bottle. The level of adrenal hormone is naturally high in the morning, progressively diminishes through the afternoon, and reaches its lowest levels in the evening. In the case of the twenty-four-hour urine sample, the doctor can determine if the total amount of hormone is high or low for the whole day, but will not know at what time of day major variations occurred. For example, a normal level for twenty-four hours might mask very high levels at one point in the day, with very low levels at another part of the day. The total for twenty-four hours would be normal, but the patient may go through half the day with excessively high levels, and the other half with excessively low.

In much the same manner, a blood cortisol level is meaningless by itself. You need to know what time of day the sample was taken. Thus, the patient's blood is drawn at a standard time of day, when there is a large sample of normal values for comparison. The standard time for taking a blood cortisol level is at eight A.M. or at four P.M.

The normal values range from 10–25 micrograms per deciliter (in the morning) and 2–10 micrograms per deciliter (in the afternoon).

Complicating this test is the fact that the blood cortisol level is dependent on the red blood cell protein molecules that carry it in the bloodstream. The amount of this protein carrier can change for a variety of reasons, which changes the level of cortisol that is measured. Abnormal estrogen levels and liver trouble also can lower the amount of this carrier protein, which will alter your test result. In addition to all this, one's level of activity can change the result of the test. Moreover, commonly used blood tests do not distinguish between protein-bound cortisol, and the unbound free form, which is more readily bioavailable. The new test for free cortisol is clearly preferable.

Stress level has a significant impact, too. Someone may have rushed to get to the lab or come from a stressful meeting at work. That would yield a different level than that of a patient who was calmly sitting in the waiting room for half an hour before the test. In addition, the conventional tests have a normal range that is very wide, so that only the most severe, out-of-range abnormalities qualify as being diagnostic of abnormal adrenal function (sound familiar?).

For these reasons, many doctors do not order adrenal tests at all. If they do, they generally focus not on cortisol, but on evaluating adrenaline levels, as did Bandura. This testing is reserved mostly for their "fight-or-flight" type patients—people whose anger and fear seem to be dominating their life.

Since adrenaline and its related compounds are known as catecholamines, testing for levels of adrenaline is also known as testing for catecholamines. It was once thought that a person who was overly stressed would display very high levels of these compounds. But the tests are hard to interpret. The phase of adrenal depletion might be adaptive (high levels), or exhaustive (low levels).

In addition, just as with the cortisol tests, the time of day, the patient's level of activity, and the exact timing of the samples during a twenty-four-hour period have sometimes proved to be daunting to the lab, the patient, and the doctor interpreting the test. Even low blood sugar triggers catecholamine release. The same difficulties for measuring twenty-four hours' worth of urinary adrenal cortex hormones would apply to measuring 24 hours worth of urinary catecholamines.

The evaluation of primary adrenal insufficiency, therefore, is best performed by giving the person a medication to stimulate the release of cortisol. The goal of this type of "challenge testing" is to measure adrenal reserve. Long before a failing adrenal gland reveals definite abnormal levels of hormone, it will go through a period of low reserve.

The way to determine the amount of adrenal reserve is to measure gland output after ACTH stimulation. The adrenal is stimulated into increased production with a quarter milligram of Cortrosyn (or some other synthetic version of ACTH), given by injection. The baseline blood cortisol is measured just prior to this injection, and the increased result is measured at the end of an hour. We believe that an increase of less than 10 micrograms, or a peak result of less than 25 micrograms, is a lowered response, thus indicating an inadequate adrenal reserve. There is not full agreement among the experts, however, about proper interpretation of either the incremental increase or the peak result.

This complicated stimulation test is much more expensive and invasive than an ordinary blood test. Moreover, it still may not tell us much at all about mild adrenal insufficiency, which could be affecting your thyroid hormone function.

Are the Alternative Options Any Better?

If conventional medicine is stymied by the adrenal system's sub-tleties, what do the alternative practitioners have to offer? They have chosen laboratories that try to assess adrenal function somewhat differently. A number of labs will do urinary measurements as described above, but instead of using twenty-four-hours' worth of urine, they use four separate samples collected at eight A.M., noon, four P.M., and midnight. Testing four different samples taken throughout the day is an attempt to obtain a more complete adrenal profile than one sample would provide. This allows a more detailed picture of the patient's daily cyclic adrenal function, and better distinguishes between the alarm phase and the exhaustion phase.

In addition to increased determinations per day, the new test measures more than cortisol levels. Also commonly tested is DHEA, a precursor to some of the other adrenal hormones. (A precursor is a chemical that is not as far along on the chemical pathway chain as the final product.) The resulting set of numbers, which some labs call the Adrenal Stress Index or ASI, can then be used to initiate and monitor therapy.

Saliva measurement is another type of test not yet considered part of a conventional adrenal workup. The determination of hormonal levels in saliva is, however, being researched for its effectiveness in assessing glandular health and balance.[3] One such saliva test is similar to the urinary ASI above. It tests four saliva samples, collected at four specific times of day (eight A.M., noon, four P.M., and midnight). Like the urinary tests just mentioned, more than cortisol levels are measured. Some saliva labs will check cortisol, DHEA, and pregnenolone. Pregnenolone, like DHEA, is a chemical precursor to many of the important adrenal hormones. The saliva measurement is a good choice because of its ease of collection and affordability, but its degree of reliability remains to be fully evaluated. It is potentially much more accurate than blood testing, because saliva tests measure only the free (bioavailable) form of the hormone.

The Great Debate on Adrenal Testing

Conventional medical doctors consider their tests useful and reliable. They regard the urine and saliva tests described above with skepticism, saying that research to prove the veracity of such testing has not yet been done.

The alternative practitioners, on the other hand, point to numbers of medical research studies in respected journals suggesting that the new technology is indeed accurate enough to be helpful, especially in diagnosing the milder versions of low adrenal function.[4] These same practitioners consider the standard medical testing overpriced and unhelpful in determining adrenal dysfunction in anyone except a severely ill patient. They say that millions of people who might have mild adrenal insufficiency, and whose lives could be improved if treated, are instead told their tests are normal. These practitioners believe that the newer urinary and saliva tests do indeed reveal mildly abnormal adrenal function.[5]

We think that the alternative tests of urine or saliva, evaluating four separate samples in a twenty-four-hour period, are the preferred choices. They seem to reveal more of what is actually occurring when a patient experiences disturbingly low points in his or her day, or when proper thyroid treatment does not go well.

However, these alternative tests are unlikely to reveal the true level of adrenal reserve. As you recall, long before routine adrenal levels run low, the gland will display decreased ability to respond well to stress ("low adrenal reserve"). In these cases a person is able to get through an ordinary day fairly well, but gets into big trouble when confronted with any stress that is out of the ordinary.

Therefore, when the alternative saliva or urine tests are normal, yet low adrenal is still suspected, our next course of action is to order the conventional medical test for low adrenal reserve (ACTH Stimulation Test, also known as Cortrosyn Stimulation Test). Testing for adrenal reserve in this fashion is similar to the definitive thyroid test of TSH reserve (TRH test) described in Step 4. These tests may be cumbersome and expensive, but proper diagnosis can lead to enormous savings in the long run.

What if *all* these adrenal tests are normal? Sometimes the prospective low-adrenal patient says, "Look, I had thyroid testing and found out that I had thyroid antibodies. Why can't I have adrenal testing to determine whether I have adrenal antibodies? Wouldn't that be useful?"

The answer is yes, it could be very useful. There is indeed a great deal of adrenal antibody illness. Some researchers estimate that as much as 70 percent of true Addison's disease (the most severe instance of adrenal failure) is due to antiadrenal antibodies. In addition, people with antibodies against their thyroid are more likely to have antibodies against their adrenals. We will explore how to deal with the autoimmune factor in greater detail in Step 9.

The Best Treatment for Low Adrenal Function

Where does all this leave us? Fortunately, the news is good. Although adrenal testing is quite complex, adrenal treatment can be quite simple.

Imagine that you have an inordinate level of anger, fear, anxiety, and stress. Suppose that you have been able to get a doctor to test you properly, and you do have mild adrenal insufficiency. One good thing to do is identify the causes of your stress and see what can be done to eliminate and/or manage them. Another is to take a small daily amount of hydrocortisone (brand name Cortef). This comes in 5 milligram tablets, and many low thyroid sufferers will find their situation improved with the simple addition of one pill daily in the morning with breakfast.

Other people with a slightly worse adrenal condition might find better improvement with one pill at breakfast and one pill at lunch. Still other people might require slightly more hormone. For them, the best way to take this kind of adrenal hormone may be four times daily, one pill at breakfast, lunch, and dinner, and one at bedtime with a small snack.

You need not increase to four times a day if a lower dose adequately improves your adrenal function. Improvement in your status can be confirmed by retesting, once you have been on medication for a month or two. You may need to take an extra dose or two of adrenal hormone temporarily, for a few days, if sudden unusual stress causes you undue fatigue. You will need even more adrenal supplementation if a respiratory infection severely diminishes your energy.

The addition of adrenal hormone to your regimen could easily result in your getting more mileage out of your thyroid hormone. In fact, many people are thereby able to reduce a high thyroid intake to a more appropriate dose.

As with thyroid hormone replacement, the literature on the subject has overemphasized the hazards of mild supplementation and minimized the enormous benefits. We want to make it clear that taking these very modest amounts of mild natural adrenal hormone, when needed, will not cause an excess of adrenal hormones in your body. Nor will you experience the side effects commonly attributed to steroids (puffy face, weakened bones and skin, high blood pressure, water retention). We're suggesting 5 milligrams of natural hydrocortisone (Cortef) one to four times per day, as opposed to 100–200 milligrams per day for treatment of severe disease. If you notice any intestinal side effects, simply stop this medicine and try something else.

Most people who are treated for inflammatory conditions of the skin, lungs, or joints are not given natural hormone. Instead, they are prescribed the much more potent, and side-effect-provoking, synthetic analogue of hydrocortisone, called prednisone. Under no circumstances are we recommending that any mildly low thyroid or low adrenal person take synthetic chemicals such as prednisone for the kind of hormone balancing we are discussing in this book.

There are also a number of nutritional products available over the counter that can be supportive or even curative of mild low adrenal function. A discussion of which natural products are most useful will be found in the next step, along with our best thoughts for other nutritional and alternative therapies to optimize your thyroid. For now, we wish you good luck for your adrenal balance.

A Self-Assessment

To explore whether there might be an adrenal component to your low thyroid function, ask yourself the following questions.

Do you have:

- Low stamina for stress, easy irritability?
- Excess mood responses after eating carbohydrates such as pasta, breads, and sugars, or marked low blood sugar or hypoglycemia?
- Chronic infections (bacterial, viral, fungal, or yeast)?
- Low blood pressure, fainting, or feeling of momentary light-headedness upon standing up?
- Chronic allergy/sensitivity to common items in environment?
- Arthritis or other chronic inflammatory response?
- "Tired but wired" feeling? Poor sleep?
- Having your best energy when others are winding down and sleeping?
- Cravings for sweets, intolerance to alcohol?
- Especially poor resistance to respiratory infections (getting them more often and being depleted when you have them)?
- Dry unhealthy skin with excess pigmentation?
- Cystic breasts (chronic cystic mastitis)?
- Difficulty recuperating from jet lag?
- Significant anxiety with depression?
- A sense of aging prematurely?

If you answered yes to four or more of these, and if you have experienced some of the difficulties outlined in this chapter, you might want to consider adrenal testing to evaluate your condition further.

The Bottom Line

- Your adrenals are two pyramid-shaped glands right above each kidney. Their job is to produce regulatory hormones, including adrenaline and cortisone, which are active during periods of stress.

- Some people who need thyroid hormone respond negatively to it, possibly indicating a coexistent low adrenal problem.
- Low adrenal, when present, should be treated along with low thyroid.
- Even for those who respond well to thyroid hormone, adrenal treatment is sometimes necessary for full improvement of the thyroid situation.
- Standard adrenal tests do not generally reveal mild adrenal dysfunction.
- The new alternative tests, evaluating four separate samples of urine or saliva, are frequently more revealing of mild insufficiency.
- Neither standard nor alternative tests are as definitive as measuring adrenal reserve with the more expensive Cortrosyn Stimulation Test (when the latter is interpreted liberally).
- When it can be determined that low adrenal should be treated, a simple and safe method is to take 5 milligrams of hydrocortisone, with food, one to four times a day.
- Hydrocortisone is a natural hormone constantly used in everyone's body for health and energy. If you are low in it, you ought to take some, especially if you are also low thyroid.

Boost Your Medication with Natural Therapies

Make your thyroid gland perform—keep it well-fed along with the rest of you.

—STEPHEN LANGER, M.D., *How to Win at Weight Loss*

So far, we have been exploring how to construct an optimal medical program for your thyroid situation. Frequently, however, even the best regimen of medicines does not relieve all low thyroid symptoms. Now, it's time to consider the fine-tuning available from a variety of nonprescription approaches.

The Best Foods to Eat If You Are Low Thyroid

Whereas some nutritionists and other natural health care providers might suggest dietary and vitamin intervention prior to any medical treatment, it is our experience that with low thyroid, the reverse is most often preferable. The prescription medication is often of initial benefit in reducing the gland's inflammation. Taking a thyroid hormone pill reduces the need for the gland to make the hormone itself. This reduction in pressure on the gland generally results in a reduction of autoimmune activity against it.

Lowering one's autoimmune activity is one of the most useful and desired results of all. A lowered autoimmune response reduces the inflammation of the gland and improves utilization of the hormone. With this initial improvement in thyroid function, your intestinal absorption of nutrients and overall body stamina are boosted. Nutritional and alternative therapies can then be employed as the adjunct that will further improve your condition, no matter what thyroid medicines you are taking.

The vast array of natural foods available today is sometimes bewildering to the consumer. Our goal here is to increase your chances of success by putting some order and clarity into a complicated and often haphazard endeavor. Most experts agree that nutritional intake is the foundation of any natural therapy program. Ironically, however, medical schools generally don't teach basic courses in nutrition. As you pursue thyroid treatment, you may find that you need to augment your doctor's information with suggestions from a good nutritionist.

Start with Food Simplicity

What we have learned about diet, vitamins, and minerals is that simplicity is the key. Try to eat the simplest of foods (preferably unrefined and untainted by chemicals that could disrupt your thyroid function). Plan your diet to be nutrient-rich, hypoallergenic, high in protein, low in fat, high in complex carbohydrates, and low in simple sugars. The high-protein aspect, especially, helps prevent autoimmune flareups. If you haven't already implemented such a diet, now is a good time to do so.

Select fresh, whole, organic foods whenever possible, meat from range-fed cattle and poultry raised on an organic diet, as well as fish from unpolluted waters (deep sea or organic fish ponds). Try buying more of your food in bulk, rather than in expensive pretty packages. Not only will you save money and generate less trash, but you will end up with more nutrients and fewer additives.

Read package labels carefully, and avoid foods with items listed on the labels that are meaningless to you. Especially avoid foods containing hard-to-pronounce chemical ingredients (which generally sound something like this: sodium bichlorohydroxy phenobiphosphoacetate). Many of these are harmful hormone blockers or hormone-mimics, which confuse the body and the immune system. If you are curious, investigate what these chemicals do by going to the library or Internet (see Step 9).

Another general recommendation is not to skip breakfast. The morning meal is an important time of day for food intake, especially for thyroid patients. Sunrise is when certain hormones are at the high point of their normal daily cycle (some hormones in the body follow daily circadian rhythms, with periodic ebbs and flows, similar to the monthly menstrual cycle). Cortisol, for example, is normally high in the early morning, lower at midday, and lowest in the evening.

What you eat in the morning, too, can set the stage for the whole day's metabolic activity. Why spend a day punctuated with fatigue and cravings for sweets, just because the orange juice, doughnuts, and coffee you ate for breakfast led to later cycles of high and low blood sugar? Far better choices would be hot cereal, or a low-fat fish or turkey patty, with whole grain toast, and a high-protein smoothie.

In general, it is a good idea to lessen your intake of dietary fat. Not only is a lower fat diet beneficial for the thyroid, but it may help to prevent other chronic conditions as well. What this means is not eating fried foods and eating minimal amounts of red meat and dairy products. While we understand that this is a departure from the standard American diet, most recent research bears out the validity of eating in this manner. The less fat in your diet, the more weight you can lose with the same caloric intake.

Since many people with thyroid disease have weight problems, it is helpful to generally reduce empty calories (desserts and fatty snack foods), while increasing exercise. These goals may seem daunting, but if you have the thyroid support described in earlier steps, it will make this task much easier than before, as untreated low thyroid can contribute to weight gain and a sluggish lifestyle.

In general, eating a healthy balanced diet of whole foods can supply most nutrients needed by the body. However, optimal eating can be challenging for people with busy lives or limited finances. In addition, not everyone has access to stores that supply organic and additive-free foods.

Also, certain people who have digestive and absorption problems may actually need far more of the essential thyroid nutrients than even high-quality food would provide. For this reason, supplementation with vitamins, minerals, and other nutrients, in pill, powder, or liquid forms, is sometimes necessary. In fact, as the quality of food decreases, the need for supplementation increases.

Please remember that food supplements generally should be taken with food, and thyroid medication pills should be taken 30 to 60 minutes earlier on an empty stomach.

Supplementation: Where to Start

Vitamins are an excellent place to start. A vitamin is a catalyst, a substance that enables other nutrients to work. It is crucial that you take a complete and high-quality multivitamin with minerals as a simple way of getting most of the nutrients we will discuss below. Most nationally advertised multiple vitamins sold in drugstores do not have the potency needed for thyroid sufferers. Generally, higher-quality vitamins are found at health food and vitamin stores. Sometimes, the highest quality supplements are those you order directly from a top company. (See Recommended Supplements for our personal vitamin recommendations.)

Let us explain one way in which vitamins can support health. Our cells and tissues are constantly subjected to highly reactive and unstable molecules known as free radicals, which are harmful by-products of normal cellular metabolism. Research is continuing to find that much of our biological damage and disease is related to injury from free radicals. They undermine our health when their numbers increase to the point of harmful accumulation, called "oxidative stress." This situation can lead to cell damage and cell death.

Antioxidant compounds help to clear these damaging chemical oxidants by protecting biomolecules from oxidative damage, especially in the muscles and brain. Some vitamins act as antioxidants by eliminating free radicals. Higher intakes of nutrient antioxidants are associated with lower levels of chronic, degenerative diseases. Antioxidants also will help the thyroid to work better because of their effect on reducing free radicals, which in turn reduces pressure on the immune and detoxification systems.

Vitamin A (retinol) is lauded for its antioxidant properties. Daily supplemental dosage for low thyroid sufferers should be between 10,000–20,000 international units (IU). This is an amount commonly found in most good multivitamin and mineral combination pills. Note that vitamin A is one of the few supplements that can become toxic at high dosages. Never take more than 25,000 IU daily.[1]

Vitamin C (L-ascorbic acid) is another vitamin that has antioxidant properties. We recommend at least 1,000 milligrams per day of vitamin C. Since most multivitamins do not contain nearly this amount, it is best to consider taking your vitamin C as an extra capsule or tablet in addition to your high-quality multivitamin with minerals. There are whole books written about the benefits of vitamin C. Suffice it to say at this point that its antioxidant properties alone make it an excellent addition for thyroid sufferers.

Vitamin E (alpha tocopherol), is yet another potent antioxidant. Generally it should not be taken in doses greater than 400 IU per day. However, if you are menopausal and having hot flashes, you may increase to 800 or 1,200 daily for excellent nonestrogen control of this uncomfortable symptom.

Next, consider adjusting your intake of B-complex to around 50 milligrams a day. In addition to this level for the entire vitamin B family, specifically adjust your intake of vitamin B_6 to about 100 milligrams daily.

Bioflavonoids are chemicals that work in conjunction with the B vitamins. They are the water soluble, brightly colored substances that often appear in fruits and vegetables as companions to vitamin C. The components of the bioflavonoids are citrin, hesperidin, rutin, flavones, and flavonals.[2] They are protective and helpful both as vitamin adjuncts and as additional antioxidants. Their ability to ease inflammation can be of great benefit for people with autoimmune thyroiditis. We recommend quercetin (250–500 milligrams daily), and pygnogenol (100–150 milligrams daily).

Minerals Crucial to Optimal Thyroid Function

More important than the vitamins, however, are minerals. These are absolutely crucial to thyroid function, especially copper, zinc, and selenium. While the research is not conclusive, it does indicate that these minerals could be instrumental in the formation and optimal utilization of thyroid hormone.

Therefore, it would make sense for your multiple vitamin and mineral combination pill to include 25 milligrams zinc, 1 milligram copper, and 100 micrograms of selenium daily. Not only is selenium now recognized as important for preventing and managing heart conditions but it has also recently been found to support the conversion of T-4 storage thyroid hormone into T-3 active thyroid hormone.

A daily intake of 100–200 micrograms of chromium helps in carbohydrate metabolism and in normalization of blood sugar fluctuations and 10–20 milligrams daily of manganese is also helpful for your thyroid status. Be sure these amounts are in your multiple vitamin. Finally, be very sure to take at least 1,200 milligrams of calcium and 400 milligrams of magnesium. Both are absolutely essential.

An excellent way to get most of the minerals that you need would be to add some sea vegetables to your diet. While not commonly consumed in the American diet, sea vegetables have gained popularity as more Asians have moved to the United States. The Japanese routinely eat wakame, nori, hijiki, dulse, arame, and kombu, which they harvest in the ocean. Kombu is basically what we call kelp, and is a fine addition to soups. Arame and hijiki, after soaking, make a tasty salad topping rich in calcium and other minerals. The thin green edible wrapper on some sushi is called nori (a preparation of seaweed) and the eating of seaweed itself is far better, safer, and more fun than taking concentrated tablets made from them. In general, it is advisable to obtain as many of your nutrients as possible from the whole food source.

Good Fats, Bad Fats

For your thyroid, add to your low-fat diet small amounts of high-quality oils, such as from fish, flaxseed, primrose, or borage. Oils provide concentrated energy to the body and help carry certain vitamins to tissues. There are good fats and bad fats, otherwise referred to as saturated and unsaturated fatty acids. Nutritionists generally advise their patients to substitute vegetable oils for animal fats, or to use unsaturated fats rather than saturated ones for cooking.

Saturated fatty acids generally come from animal sources; unsaturated from plants. Plant oils contain monounsaturated fats, diunsaturated fats, and polyunsaturated fats, all in varying percentages depending on the particular plant source in question. The most favorable mix of these varying kinds of fatty acids is found in olive oil, which has a large amount of monounsaturated fats.

The worst kinds of fats are the plant oils that have been hydrogenated (artificially saturated with hydrogen) so as to be more solid at room temperature. These so-called trans-fats are the basis of margarine and many oils used in fast-food products, as well as most commercial peanut butters. They are absolutely to be avoided.

Supplements containing specific fats can be purchased as pills from local health food or vitamin stores. They can provide you with the right essential fatty acids (EFAs) for optimal thyroid function and decreased autoimmune attacks. Two essential fatty acids must be consumed orally because they cannot be manufactured in our bodies: linoleic and linolenic. Some researchers recommend 250–500 milligrams daily of the omega-6 (linoleic) variety, also called GLA, and 500–1,000 milligrams of the omega-3 (linolenic) fatty acids, also known as EPA.

One good source of both of these essential fatty acids is flaxseed oil, of which you can take two teaspoons daily. Even better would be to grind up two tablespoons of the whole flaxseeds (you can use a coffee bean grinder) and sprinkle immediately over cereal. Ground flaxseeds contain more nutrients than the oil, as well as increased fiber.[3]

Amino acids comprise a less-known category of nutritional supplements. These are the basic building blocks of all proteins. Three or more amino acids joined together form a peptide. Several peptides join to form a polypeptide. An extremely long polypeptide, which is then folded into a complex configuration, forms what we call protein. Some large polypeptides are neurotransmitters and some small proteins, such as insulin, are important hormones. Protein is also the major component of skin, tendon, and muscle.

An exception to the rule that a great many amino acids linked together form hormones and neurotransmitters is the case of the single amino acid, tyrosine. It is the basis for both kinds of thyroid hormone, as well as for adrenaline and noradrenaline. T-3 and T-4 are made of three or four atoms respectively of iodine attached to the tyrosine molecule. Adrenaline and noradrenaline are simply tyrosine with some very minor chemical additions to its ring and tail structure.

Increased amounts of the amino acid tyrosine are therefore a sensible recommendation for actual and potential thyroid sufferers. A very good way to make sure you are getting adequate tyrosine and improving overall thyroid function in general is to take a small amount of a mixture of individual amino acids, including tyrosine, every day (see Recommended Supplements).

Additional individual supplementation with the amino acid glutamine can confer a variety of benefits in everything from brain function to better digestion. For dose amounts, and more information about the marvelous benefits of glutamine amino acid support, we suggest *The Diet Cure* by Julia Ross[4] (see Further Reading).

A convenient way to get your amino acids and trace minerals would be through freeze-dried food powders. These are mixtures of dried algae and green vegetables. Some people add a small amount of this concentrated supplement to their orange juice or morning shake, along with flaxseed oil and protein powder for enhanced energy.

A morning shake can be a convenient and quick way to help satisfy one's energy needs. Karilee starts each day with a shake that mixes rice milk, protein powder, powdered vitamins, freeze-dried greens, and a tablespoon of flaxseed oil. She likes to flavor it with carob powder.

Natural Glandular Support

Another category of supplementation is that of the natural glandulars. These are considered nutritional products, but their use borders on the medicinal. They are generally tablets, occasionally capsules, of freeze-dried purified animal glands, with their associated hormones removed. This removal of active ingredients is why the glandulars can be sold over the counter at vitamin and health stores.

You might try a 100 percent natural treatment for borderline low thyroid, using only thyroid glandular tablets and the nutritional supplements outlined above. Even though thyroid glandular contains no active T-3 or T-4 (although perhaps a little is left in, similar to the amount of caffeine remaining in decaffeinated coffee), the ingestion of glandulars can result in surprisingly good benefits for many people.

Consider the case of Mary. She maintained an attitude of "natural" in her approach to health. The idea of taking prescription medicine, even the natural Armour thyroid, was absolutely against her belief system. By the time she turned forty-two, however her hypothyroidism had reached the point that simple nutritional supplementation of vitamins and minerals was no longer sufficient for her needs. She added two tablets (130 milligrams each) twice daily of a pure thyroid glandular.

Within ten days, Mary's symptoms of dry skin, hair loss, and chilliness had lessened. Other people generally find that the glandulars take longer than this to demonstrate their effectiveness, and not everyone who tries them experiences significant benefit. We recommend a very careful approach to the glandular products. If you try the glandulars for a couple of months with no improvement, it would then be time to discontinue their use. Certain people who do not benefit from the glandulars seem to have an unassailable need for actual thyroid hormone. Conversely, some people who are already taking actual thyroid hormone (synthetic type) benefit from adding glandular to it. Once again, the proof is in the patient.

This is also true for adrenal glandulars. As you learned in Step 7, adrenal support for your thyroid situation is frequently worth considering. The safest approach to such support may be taking the milder over-the-counter adrenal glandulars, rather than the stronger prescription medicine. When using adrenal glandular, however, consider starting with one tablet every other day. Then, after one week, increase to one tablet daily; after another week, go to one or two tablets twice a day. If after two months on this latter regimen you have not noticed any benefit, then you might best drop the glandular and consider the stronger prescription medicine.

Also, keep in mind that the adrenal gland has two separate outputs—cortisone and adrenaline. You may need only the cortisone supplementation, but the glandular product may augment both, creating a problem for you. This is possibly the reason many low adrenal patients feel too "speedy" on adrenal glandular supplementation.

If the glandular you try seems too stimulating, and you don't want prescription medicine, then other over-the-counter items are available for adrenal support. These include pregnenolone and DHEA, which are both considered to be precursors to other steroid hormones. Licorice root extract stimulates production and utilization of adrenal hormones. Phosphatidyl serene helps reduce the overproduction of adrenal hormones seen in the adaptive phase of adrenal gland exhaustion.

Please secure the assistance of a knowledgeable nutritionist or natural medicine practitioner before adding these substances to your thyroid program. Their benefits can be great, but they are strong medicines in their own right.

Along the same lines, low thyroid sufferers who need additional female hormone balance might well consider taking glandular ovary, or Mexican yam products, also sold at most health food stores. Although these and other female hormone boosters can be wonderfully helpful, we urge you to secure expert guidance before incorporating them into your thyroid program.

Herbal Medicines: Nature's Grand Pharmacy

Many of today's most commonly used medicines had their origin long ago in herbal remedies. Prior to pharmacies, patients followed the advice of apothecaries who prepared foxglove leaf (contains digitalis, used to treat heart ailments today), willow bark (source of aspirin), and valerian root (a sedative whose name was the inspiration for the brand name Valium).

Herbs can be useful in easing many of the individual symptoms of low thyroid. Calendula flower cream and castor oil are handy for severely dry skin. Teas of valerian, scullcap, passion flower, and hops are great for insomnia. Black cohosh has been helpful for women's menopausal difficulties, but should not be used by pregnant women. A popular and useful product called Remifemin is composed mainly of black cohosh. The herbal substance Vitex is a good stimulant for sluggish estrogen production. Even more balancing overall is the well-known Chinese medicine formula of several female-friendly herbs, called Two Immortals.

We must caution you about stimulant herbs such as ma huang (also known as ephedra), guarana, and gotu kola. These plant substances have an adrenaline-like effect on the body. Just as with caffeine and other chemical stimulants, they are not a good answer for low thyroid.

Here's one example. A thirty-seven-year-old with low-thyroid came from another clinic to see us for treatment of severe fatigue. Despite a good thyroid hormone regimen, he was only able to get to and from work and had no energy for exercise or social life. On the first visit, he told us, "Besides my medication, which helped me get back on the job, I'm taking a lot of supplements, but they are not working."

When we asked what supplements he was taking, he said, "Lots of guarana and ma huang." There may be nothing wrong with these herbal energy boosters in the short run, but if an underlying problem is not addressed, they will only help temporarily. These energy stimulants do not address the specific thyroid problem, per se. They are not the same as taking other glandular and herbal remedies specifically for improving thyroid function. Instead, they are a general and temporary body booster, like caffeine.

Just as you may feel an energy surge by ingesting caffeine or sugar but eventually you will rebound and feel more lethargic than before, so it goes when you take general herbal stimulants to treat the specific fatigue of low thyroid. The underlying reason for your low energy has not been addressed, so low energy continues.

As it turned out, we were able to pinpoint a mineral deficiency in this particular patient using a simple lab test of his blood and urine. He was prescribed a good multimineral product with extra potassium and chromium. He soon felt much better and eventually had energy to spare.

Low thyroid is generally not well addressed by the most commonly used herbs. Other less common herbal medicines do, however, seem to have a direct effect on boosting thyroid hormone.

Several interesting reports describe the salutary effects of the herb ashwagandha, whose Latin name is *Withania somnifera*.[5] An aqueous extract of the plant root had a stimulatory effect on both T-3 and T-4 thyroid hormone levels in laboratory animals. In fact, the increase in T-4 was quite dramatic. This product is now therapeutically available, and it does show promise. The main additional herb we recommend is milk thistle (silymarin), 300 milligrams daily, as an excellent additional antioxidant.

Supplement Summary

Over-the-counter nutritional items comprise an important part of your thyroid program. Deciding what to take is a very individualized process, and dosage strength is not well regulated. Because of the wide variation in content and changing quality of natural thyroid-related products, we recommend that you consult our thyroid information/treatment clearinghouse by checking our website (www.thyroidpower.com), or by calling toll-free 1-866-GoThyRx (1-866-468-4979).

What to Avoid

Removing harmful items from your inner and outer environments is one of the most important aspects of a thyroid-promoting lifestyle. These can include harmful food additives and types of food that detract from thyroid function. Most deleterious are the everyday legal drugs: caffeine, alcohol, tobacco, and sugar. Nicotine especially impairs the conversion of T-3 from T-4. The other items detract from thyroid function more indirectly.

Reducing these irritating substances can be one of the most difficult tasks a thyroid-compromised person has to face. Many people with undiagnosed low thyroid have learned to rely on these substances for the temporary energy boost they provide. Nevertheless, we urge you to take whatever steps might be necessary. For some people, this amounts to a major lifestyle change that requires socializing with a different crowd of people and perhaps even attending twelve-step recovery groups. How important is your long-term health and the quality of your daily life? We hope you will find whatever support is needed for your optimal recovery.

Specific Food Concerns

Thyroid sufferers do best to avoid foods containing compounds known to disrupt thyroid function. Some of these are known as goitrogens because their continued ingestion can result in a goiter, or a swelling of the thyroid gland. Eating large quantities of foods such as walnuts, almonds, sorghum, peanuts, pine nuts, millet, and cassava (tapioca) can result in the release of substances that may form goitrogens in the body, thereby impairing the thyroid gland.

In addition, certain nutritional authorities also suggest avoiding high intake of the otherwise very nutritious Brussels sprouts, cauliflower, cabbage, broccoli, turnips, mustard greens, spinach, and rutabaga, due to their interference with normal thyroid function. It may be advisable to limit intake of these foods to one serving per day. Since cooking usually neutralizes goitrogens in these foods, be sure that if you do eat any of them, you do so after adequate cooking.

Another major food category to consider is soy. Many health-oriented diets recommend eating several servings a day of various soy products. Certainly for vegetarians, soy is a major source of protein. However, people with low thyroid may want to limit their intake and eat only cooked soy products. As with the vegetables mentioned above, cooking helps neutralize the goitrogens.

A number of studies have suggested a link between heavy soy ingestion and thyroid autoimmunity or goiter, both in infants on soy formula and in adults eating soy foods. In adults, soy products appear to elevate T-4 without modifying T-3, changing this ratio in an important, predictable way. The elevation of T-4, without a corresponding elevation of T-3, not only results in weight gain but also in impaired thyroid function generally.

Other researchers have found a correlation between soy's plant-derived estrogens and mild disruption of thyroid activity. A compound found in soy, called genistein, apparently blocks the action of iodine and tyrosine in the production of thyroid hormone. This effect is dose-related. In other words, if the amount you eat of this otherwise healthy food is modest, then your thyroid will not be bothered.

According to Daniel R. Doerge, Ph.D., researcher at the FDA's National Center for Toxicology: "I don't think you can get into trouble [with your thyroid] if you eat a few soy foods within the bounds of a balanced diet. I see substantial risk from taking soy supplements or eating huge amounts of soy foods for their putative disease-preventing value."[6]

So, what is a modest amount? We recommend that thyroid sufferers limit their intake to one serving of soy each day. One serving of tofu would be four ounces; one serving of soy milk is eight ounces. One serving of soy sauce or miso would be two teaspoons.

For most people on a standard American diet, it would be a grand step in the right direction to introduce some soy products in place of fatty meats. The small amount of soy foods that the average person is likely to eat is in no way problematic to their thyroid. The admonishment to limit intake is given largely for the benefit of people who have substituted soy for animal products and rely solely on vegetarian sources for their protein. Once again, balance is the key.

Fluoridated Water: A Bad Idea Whose Time Has Passed

We believe that the thyroid epidemic could be due, in large part, to the bombardment of our collective thyroid glands by chemicals that are presently or were once considered to be helpful. If you have a thyroid problem, avoiding fluoride may be a good preventive health measure for you. Fluoride is added routinely to toothpaste to prevent tooth decay. Moreover, it is routinely being added to public drinking water for the same purpose.

Yet, this same substance, currently touted as harmless enough to be put into the water supply, has been used in the past as a powerful medication to slow down overactive thyroid activity.[7] Because of the development of newer antithyroid medicines, including propyl-thiouracil (PTU) and methimazole (Tapazole), fluoride has not been used to treat hyperthyroidism for many decades.

The original research that suggested fluoride's benefit to teeth was done with pharmaceutical grade sodium fluoride. This is *not* what is being added to drinking water today. Instead, 90 percent of fluoridated communities use waste products primarily from the phosphate fertilizer and aluminum industries. There has been *no* water safety research done on these chemicals.

John Lee, M.D., long-time practicing physician, author, and lecturer, has reported that in his many years of observations, vulnerable people can be either hypothyroid or normal in thyroid function, depending on whether or not they live in fluoridated communities. In fact, he has seen patients who have gone in and out of hypothyroidism, solely related to their movement to and from cities with fluoride added to the water.

As health professionals, we feel a moral obligation to share our growing concern about the fluoridation issue. In addition to fluoride's possible thyroid-lowering effect on the population at large, it has come to our attention that there may well be other even more devastating effects.

A search of the history of fluoridation focusing on the late 1940s, the time of its initial introduction into drinking water, reveals that there appears to have been a connection between the special interests of a large industry and the public policy that favored any city's decision to fluoridate the local water supply. For those interested in more details, we have compiled a listing of research articles and websites. The information may astound you (see Fluoride Facts). It certainly caught us by surprise.

Of major interest to us is the statement in a release dated July 2, 1997 from the National Treasury Employees Union, Chapter 280, (formerly NFFE, Local 2056), which represents 1,500 scientists, engineers, lawyers, and other professionals at the Environmental Protection Agency headquarters in Washington, D.C. This statement reads: "Our members' review of the body of evidence over the last eleven years, including animal and human epidemiology studies, indicates a causal link between fluoride/fluoridation and cancer, genetic damage, neurological impairment, and bone pathology." If fluoride is now suspected of causing these deleterious effects, and also has been used in the past as medication to slow thyroid function, why does our government still support the policy of adding it to our drinking water?

Notably, in 1990 the Environmental Protection Agency fired the Office of Drinking Water's chief toxicologist, Dr. William Marcus, for refusing to remain silent on the fluoride risk issues, particularly the cancer risk. Dr. Marcus sued for reinstatement and won. These events teach us that we cannot always rely on long-standing government policy. We must question, and seek the facts, rather than wait until too much damage has been done.

Even the early research done to support the initial addition of fluoride into drinking water was questionable. For example, in 1945 the U.S. Public Health Service began to add sodium fluoride to the drinking water in Grand Rapids, Michigan, the first city in the United States to fluoridate. Grand Rapids was supposed to serve as the test city. Its dental decay rates were to be compared with those of Muskegon, Michigan, which was nonfluoridated. After ten years, it was supposed to be determined if fluoride was safe and effective. Amazingly, this "research" was to be performed on an entire city, rather than by using a voluntary sample group initially. More strange was what occurred before the study was completed.

As stated by John Yiamouyiannis, Ph.D., in his book *Fluoride: The Aging Factor:*

> In 1950, long before any studies had been completed to determine whether the addition of fluoride to the public water supplies was a safe and effective means of reducing tooth decay, the Public Health Service and the American Dental Association endorsed fluoridation. Within a short time thereafter, Muskegon, the control city in the Grand Rapids study, was fluoridated . . . These endorsements effectively overshadowed the fact that the tooth decay rate in non-fluoridated Muskegon had decreased about as much as in fluoridated Grand Rapids—and that fluoridation was ineffective in reducing decay in permanent teeth.[8]

Other cities then began to fluoridate. Moreover, they started to substitute different fluoride products for sodium fluoride. The substitutes were sodium silicofluoride products, primarily hydrofluosilicic acid, from the fertilizer and aluminum industries. In 1950, the Public Health Service gave its blessing to the use of these alternate sources of fluoride, without having researched them.

At that time, no one had any data on the long-term detrimental health effects of the silicofluorides. The EPA admits it still does not have any such data, nor does the Center for Disease Control (CDC), the agency responsible for promoting water fluoridation.

According to Dartmouth researcher Myron J. Coplan, co-author of the famous Dartmouth Study,[9] about 90 percent of all "fluoride adjusted" water today is treated with a silicofluoride chemical. So, whereas laboratory research was initially performed on sodium fluoride, within a few years, other "similar" products were substituted, without adequate study.

Masters and Coplan have found an association between the use of silicofluorides and the uptake of lead in young children. In addition, fluoride poisoning itself is indeed possible. According to the National Library of Medicine's Toxnet database, hydrofluosilicic acid is classified as a toxic waste product in certain concentrations (and yes, there have been "accidental poisonings" in community water supplies since this practice was introduced). It is considered to be a fairly strong acid, capable of attacking glass and stoneware. The concentration put into our water supply may not be toxic initially, but who is monitoring the long-term accumulation and total intake from multiple other sources such as dental treatments and the use of fluoride toothpaste at home?

The Department of Transportation guidelines for this product say "TOXIC: inhalation, ingestion, or skin contact may cause severe injury or death." (See Fluoride Facts for websites about fluoride toxicity.) The website information also reveals that workers handling such dangerous substances should be supplied with eye and face protection, respiratory protective equipment, protective clothing, and foot and leg protection, as well as possibly needing to use a barrier cream. Isn't it strange how the general public doesn't always hear of these hazards?

Only 2 percent of Europe fluoridates, and less than 5 percent of the world's population drinks fluoridated water. Large studies in the United States and New Zealand have shown little or no difference in the teeth of children living in fluoridated and nonfluoridated communities, except for the disturbing finding that communities with fluoridation have more cases of dental fluorosis (a defect of tooth enamel, resulting in mottling of teeth).

Today, more than fifty years after the introduction of fluoride, a growing debate is emerging across the United States, and throughout the world, with regard to fluoridation. A number of countries, including India, Japan, Finland, Denmark, Sweden, and Holland, have either rejected or banned the addition of this industrial waste product to community drinking water supplies.

People opposed to water fluoridation also express concern about the government's power to put any substance in the community drinking water without the express consent of all individuals affected. According to antifluoridationists, this power sets a dangerous precedent, and contradicts an individual's right to choose what he or she ingests. Some people feel very strongly that the public is being "mass medicated"—without its consent. After all, the first occurrence of fluoridated drinking water on Earth was found in Germany's Nazi prison camps. Their reason for medicating the water was to force inmates into calm submission.

Fluoride opponents are suggesting that dentists focus their efforts on providing sodium fluoride tablets or treatments to all people who want it, or need it, including the poor, rather than dumping it into the water we all use. Over 99 percent of it, paid for by taxes, ends up on our lawns and in swimming pools and rivers, rather than on our teeth. Still, the amount we absorb accumulates as we shower, bathe, and swim in it. Since the fluoride in drinking water may also be in our juices, beers, wines, and other drinks, there is no way to know how much we're ingesting, but we do know how much is too much. (Five milligrams per day will lower thyroid function and over time lead to skeletal fluorosis.)

We are suggesting—especially during such a chaotic time in the history of medicine—that it is up to each health consumer to vigorously guard his or her health—literally. Guard it with your life. Keep an open mind, review the data, listen to the concerns of others in your community, consider becoming involved in health issues of concern, and vote.

Be certain that your voice is heard and that all decisions are guided by the ethical principle to which physicians, nurses, and other health care professionals have pledged to adhere. "Above all, do no harm." We believe that if we don't know whether doing something is good or harmful, we are obligated to choose the most conservative path: the one less likely to do harm. For more information about possible cancer connections, decreased IQ in children, and other fluoride-related concerns and studies, see Fluoride Facts (see Resources for companies that will mail you excellent equipment for eliminating fluoride from your drinking and bathing water). For those severely affected, distillation and reverse osmosis water treatment may offer great relief.

What About Fluoridated Toothpaste?

We recommend that anyone with low thyroid use toothpaste without fluoride. It is available, but you will have to do some careful shopping to find it. Even many of the "natural" toothpaste products at health food stores contain fluoride.

Discuss your personal concerns and needs with your dentist if you have a thyroid problem. Do not allow your children to be treated with fluoride. Do your best to explore other options. We are not convinced that teeth are more important than overall health. Find a dentist who will help you encourage your children to avoid sweets and brush and floss regularly, and who is respectful of your wishes and beliefs.

A Surprising Nutrient to Avoid

One other supposedly friendly item for autoimmune thyroid people to avoid may surprise you. It is iodine, a substance that most people believe is good for thyroid function. Iodine is indeed a major constituent of thyroid hormone. In fact, worldwide, the enormous problem of low thyroid is basically one of iodine deficiency, though this is hardly the case in the United States. Even in the so-called "Midwest goiter belt" (an area of the United States where, early in the twentieth century, so many people suffered from goiter that it earned that demographic definition), the problem has been handled by the addition of iodine to commonly eaten foods such as table salt.

People who live on or near the coasts usually do not have an iodine deficiency, perhaps because of the abundant iodine in the soil where local food is grown and in the seafood they eat. Nevertheless, some practitioners constantly recommend iodine supplementation for patients with autoimmune low thyroid. We recommend that people in the United States should be cautious of this older advice.

Iodine is a double-edged sword for thyroid sufferers. More than adequate amounts (i.e., anything more than the standard 150 micrograms in a multivitamin-mineral combination), may further irritate and inflame an already ailing thyroid gland. If you are already on thyroid hormone, you might want to take a multivitamin without any additional iodine.

How does excess iodine harm the thyroid system? A high amount of iodine in the body becomes concentrated in the thyroid gland, in the hormone precursor protein called thyroglobulin. A high amount of iodinated thyroglobulin triggers the autoimmune response. An extreme form of this scenario would be a person with mild autoimmune thyroiditis, deciding on ill advice to take extra iodine. Before long the excessively irritated thyroid gland becomes inflamed and dysfunctional.

In fact, some scientists now suggest that part of the reason for the present epidemic of low thyroid in the United States may be the high amount of iodine in many people's diets. Not surprisingly, we may have gone too far in attempting to eliminate goiters in small regions by adding iodine to the entire country's salt.

In much the same way, we may have gone too far in attempting to eliminate rampant tooth decay in a particular subpopulation by putting extra fluoride in everyone's drinking water. These overzealous global responses may not be merited in future similar situations. As a human community, we must exert our greatest creativity toward finding solutions that help those in need, without creating further problems for others.

Fast food, canned food, and prepackaged food all contain significant amounts of salt, mostly the iodized kind. People who regularly eat this kind of food, and those who frequent restaurants as well, could be consuming between 8 and 10 grams of salt a day. At 70 micrograms of iodine per gram of salt, this could amount to 560–700 micrograms daily intake, more than four times the recommended daily allowance.

Not only is this too much for people genetically prone to autoimmune thyroid disease, but, in addition, many people also eat lobster, crab, and shellfish, all of which are rich in iodine. All of this, in our view, adds up to a clear overdose of iodine for many at-risk individuals. To avoid excessive iodine intake, do your best to avoid iodized salt, unless you live in goiter-endemic areas, such as the Great Lakes region and unless you never consume seafood, sushi, or vitamins that contain iodine.

What about the majority of the population that is *not* genetically prone to autoimmune thyroid disease? Should they be trying to avoid iodine as well? The answer is *no*. The worldwide tragedy of iodine deficiency disease is still enough of a threat to warrant continued iodine supplementation for the "average" person.

Sweet but Dangerous?

One final note about what to avoid. The sugar substitutes Equal and NutraSweet may seem innocent enough, but they could be problematic for your metabolism. They contain an amino-acid-related compound called aspartame. We do not at all recommend it for thyroid sufferers.

People with autoimmune thyroid are generally more allergic than

the average person, and even the average person sometimes has sensitivity to this artificial compound. Aspartame's ingredients compete
with normal amino acid metabolism, specifically blocking the conversion of tryptophan into the neurotransmitter serotonin. Remember that serotonin is one of the mood-enhancing, "feel-good"
chemicals of the brain. We want to keep those chemicals flowing.

We want you to keep all your healthy chemicals flowing. Use your
body as a laboratory to find out for yourself which foods serve as your
best fuel and which supplements agree with your specific constitution. Finally, identify which items are best to avoid so that you may
more fully enjoy your health journey.

The Bottom Line

- Even a great medical regimen may need additional help.
- Healthier food may be your best additional medicine, and fast
  food your worst poison (see Food Choices).
- Cover more of the bases with specific thyroid-boosting supplements (see Recommended Supplements chart).
- An easy way to cover many bases at once is with a high-
  quality combination vitamin and mineral pill taken once
  daily.
- What to avoid may be just as important as what to ingest.
  Thyroid function improves with less caffeine, alcohol,
  tobacco, and sugar.
- Specifically avoid extra large intake of thyroid-blocking foods,
  such as soy and certain cruciferous vegetables.

Improve the Underlying Autoimmune Condition

In reality, about 25% of individuals do seem to have . . . the unfortunate capacity to make antibodies to fragments of some of their own body cells.

—LAWRENCE C. WOOD, M.D., *Your Thyroid*

The structure of normal thyroid tissue, under a microscope, is one of the most beautiful and harmonious in the body. The cells are arranged like a circle of houses around a central lake. Multiple lakes, each with its own circle of cells, form an attractive geometric design. Inside each lake is colloid, a colorful substance able to hold hormone-assembly materials within it, the same way that Jell-O can hold peaches. Medical students are in awe of the beauty of this tissue.

When antibodies and infiltrating white blood cells attack this harmonious picture, the symmetrical architecture of the houses and lakes becomes tangled. Some of the cells shrivel, others disappear. The blood vessels become thin and inflamed. The perfectly round iridescent lakes become jagged and drained of their luminosity. Frequently they vanish entirely. In severe cases, the tissue resembles the twisted aftermath of a hurricane or tornado. A gland that has been attacked in this way can hardly produce the right amount, or right kind, of thyroid hormone. What causes this attack, and what can you do about it?

If the previous eight steps have helped you regain 90 percent or more of your true healthy self, then you may not have to do anything further about the autoimmune issue. If, on the other hand, you would like to pursue further benefit in your thyroid status, tackling the autoimmune issue is your next step.

The Mystery of Autoimmune Attack

Current medical science does not provide easy solutions for people with autoimmune low energy. It is not simply that the underlying reason for the low energy is missed, though this is often the case. Even when the problem is diagnosed properly, the treatment frequently falls short.

In autoimmune conditions, the whole body is involved, rather than just the organ that has been attacked. The damaged organ, in this case the thyroid, is referred to as the target-organ. This is medical lingo for the part that displays the symptoms of the total body autoimmune situation. Interventions are generally directed only at the target-organ, and not the source of the problem, which is the entire immune system.

Total Body Immunity

Taking hormones and vitamins for autoimmune low thyroid is similar to taking nose drops or eye drops for hay fever. The drops can help the symptoms but can never fully address the cause of the problem.

Thyroid doctors do not generally address the immune system problem because almost every standard medicine in the conventional medical arsenal is ineffective for autoimmunity. Recently developed immune-boosting medicines are not appropriate when the immune system is already in autoimmune overdrive. Even the new immune-modulator drugs such as Paxone and Avonex are not used for thyroiditis. Unfortunately, doctors simply do not have a pill that will directly reduce the autoimmune component of low thyroid.

However, many nondrug approaches offer substantial promise. Before using them, you need a clear sense of what is causing your particular version of the illness.

Multiple Triggers of the Autoimmune Event

A person's tendency for the autoimmune reaction is in part genetic. There is presently no way to do much about that, except to choose your ancestors more carefully! We can, however, learn ways to reduce the factors that trigger the autoimmune tendency into a full-blown autoimmune attack.

One trigger is age. Some people's internal time clock goes off, and their autoimmune thyroiditis gets triggered. This can occur at any age, for no apparent reason, without another precipitating event. On the other hand, some women's thyroiditis is triggered by fluctuations in their female hormone levels, specifically at the unsettled times of puberty or menopause.

Other women find that the end of pregnancy is a trigger. This response is named postpartum thyroiditis. Many women who are diagnosed with postpartum depression, or postpartum low energy, actually have autoimmune inflammation of the thyroid gland.

Other triggers that have been described range from accidents, operations, and severe infections, to bulimia, crash dieting, and major changes in lifestyle.[1] A few of our patients suffered from specific trauma to the neck (especially whiplash), which apparently triggered their long-term thyroid inflammation. Scientists believe that the antibody inflammation gets started secondary to cell destruction from some other mechanism. This other mechanism can cause irritation and damage to the thyroid cells through the effects of outside chemicals, free radicals, food allergy, and perhaps other irritants.

Even certain medicines can kick it off. Recall from Step 8 that a surprisingly destructive nutrient is iodine. While small amounts of iodine are absolutely necessary for thyroid health, large amounts can trigger the autoimmune response. Iodinated medications and dyes used for X ray contrast are common culprits. For example, the iodine-containing heart medicine amiodarone causes low thyroid in 20 percent of the people who take it.[2] Once triggered, the low thyroid activity can either resolve spontaneously or persist for many years.

Other medicines can trigger the autoimmune illness called lupus. Silica is known to cause autoimmunity in quartz miners. Years ago in Spain, vinyl chloride–tainted olive oil caused many thousands of people to contract the rare autoimmune illness scleroderma. Today, some medical centers even have experts in chemical-caused autoimmunity.

It is even possible for severe stress alone to be a trigger. This should not be totally surprising, when considering the number of documented incidents in which stress has been shown to affect immune function. It may be part of the genetic makeup of certain individuals to be anxious and worried, which in itself predisposes them to this kind of triggering effect.

Fortunately, this is one genetic tendency where intervention has been successful. You may not be able to change your genetic makeup, but you can learn to be less stressed by life events, reducing the likelihood of triggering further autoimmune difficulty. We will present several good stress-management strategies in the section below, where we discuss immediate actions you can take.

Environmental Pollution—the Chemical Triggers

We believe the thyroid epidemic is due in large part to excess chemicals in food, air, and water, confusing and stressing our immune system. This amazing collection of cells and tissues, which exists for our protection, appears to be baffled and threatened by the insult of so many different chemicals bombarding us. As the number of immune-sensitizing chemicals proliferates in our environment, we are seeing an increased incidence of autoimmune illness.

The process of chemicals triggering autoimmune low thyroid falls into the category of what is called hormone-disruption. In *Our Stolen Future*,[3] their fabulous book on the international chemical health problem, Colburn, Dumanosky, and Myers reveal that the delicate thyroid hormone balance is one of the most frequent targets for synthetic chemicals.

No one knows for sure, but here is how these hormone-disruptors may affect thyroid via the immune process. The success of the immune system in defending our body, but not attacking it, relies on an incredibly complex and intricately balanced network of billions of specialized cells. Their elaborate and dynamic regulatory network has a sensitive system of hormonal checks and balances. It normally produces an immune response that is prompt, effective, and self-limiting.

In the presence of hormone disruptors, however, the reverse may be the case. A drawn-out, ineffective, and not self-limited immune response could easily go even more awry. The lymphocytes could become disorganized, and the antibody levels unbalanced. The now confused system could begin to overreact, like a disturbed hornets' nest. The immune cells might then begin to attack a healthy tissue, acting on the false notion that they detect a foreign invader. The result could trigger one's latent genetic autoimmune tendency into a full-blown autoimmune response.

The number of hormone disruptors is astounding. Worldwide, this problem seems mainly due to pesticides (herbicides, fungicides, insecticides, nematocides) constantly being released into the environment, occasionally hundreds to thousands of tons at a time. Many of them contain PCBs (polychlorinated biphenyls, common in insecticides), and dioxins (frequently found in common herbicides and especially Agent Orange).

There are over 200 compounds classified as PCBs, and 80 different dioxins. Both types of compounds have a wide variety of documented disruptive effects. On the other hand, most of the tens of thousands of other synthetic chemicals created and dumped into the environment in the past forty years have not been well studied. In fact, many of the best-known cases of endocrine disruptors were discovered by accident.

Environmental writer Marla Cone has gathered and summarized a great deal of the current thinking related to these immune-provoking pollutants. In an article for the *Los Angeles Times,* she made it clear that ". . . autoimmune diseases have increased internationally, and seem to have popped up in extraordinary clusters in communities tainted with toxic chemicals."[4] Careful investigation allowed her to list common polluting chemicals and the various autoimmune conditions caused by these chemicals. The PCBs, some of the most ubiquitous, seem to be responsible for many of the autoimmune thyroid problems. Cone noted that the closer people live to pollution sources, the higher their auto-antibodies, a measurement of the severity of the immune cells' attack on healthy tissues.

There is more about PCBs and thyroid in the remarkable volume, *Hormonal Chaos*[5] by Sheldon Krimsky, a professor of Urban and Environmental Policy. Dr. Krimsky eloquently details the staggering problem posed by the large number of hormone disruptors in our environment.

The chemical triggering of autoimmune low thyroid is only part of what is called the environmental endocrine hypothesis. This idea currently sits somewhere between theory and fact, depending upon who tells the story. For nonbelievers in this hormone-disruptor connection, no number of citations of scientific studies would be sufficient to convince them. For the believers, none is necessary. The future of the hypothesis is currently in the hands of government officials and their science advisers, all daunted by the potentially overwhelming magnitude of the problem.

Dozens of synthetic chemicals that we willingly use every day, ranging from dish soap to deodorant, could be contributing to the chronic illnesses we face. Hormone disruption has emerged as one of the top research priorities of the Environmental Protection Agency. One of its recent tasks has been to attempt to systematically check the 15,000 most common pesticides, solvents, and other synthetic compounds to see which ones are hormonally active. Some seem to cause low thyroid through direct toxicity, rather than by the autoimmune route.

Choose your side carefully in this debate. Your health, and the quality of your life, may depend on it. Recall from Step 1 that it took almost two thousand years to fully understand the cause of a large epidemic facing the Romans. You may not want to wait until all the answers are in before taking sensible precautionary actions against the present thyroid epidemic.

Sensible and Immediate Actions to Take

Someday, science may be able to correct the genetic defect that makes thyroid sufferers so susceptible to internal and environmental triggers. Until then, what can a person do to "call off the dogs," to lessen the chances that an overzealous immune system will attack one's own thyroid gland?

The most important thing is to live your life more chemical free and immune friendly. Our focus in this step is not the question of tissue "toxicity," but one of immune "sensitivity." Even smaller amounts than would be toxic can be very sensitizing to your delicate immune system. Having offered this warning, let us now examine how your life can be less polluted and more chemical free.

Beginning Steps

You might start reading household product labels the same way that you read food labels and make efforts to decrease the amount of nasty-sounding ingredients in your shampoos, detergents, and toothpaste. The next thing to do is look closely at your life and habits. Just what, other than chemicals, is most likely to be annoying your immune system?

It might be exposure to a particular inhaled irritant. It might be related to eating allergy-provoking food such as corn or chocolate. It could even be the proximity of a particular pet that always makes you sneeze. Stressing your immune system by constant exposure to something you know you are allergic to will just make the autoimmune low thyroid situation worse.

Water Filtration

Another way to protect yourself against immune sensitizers and endocrine disruptors is to use a water purifying system in your home and workplace. The filters readily available in neighborhood stores are designed primarily to remove bacteria, microorganisms, and unpleasant taste or odor. They may not remove the synthetic chemicals that can sensitize the immune system or alter hormone function.

The simplest, most affordable water filter to remove synthetic chemicals is a carbon block filter. Also, as noted in Step 8, it is important to decrease your fluoride exposure. Removing fluoride requires the more comprehensive treatment of reverse-osmosis or distillation (see Resources).

Don't assume that the water source used for expensive bottled water is any better than the source used for your tap water. Most bottled water is unregulated, and it sits for long periods of time in containers that may leach plastic-related compounds into the water itself (especially when left in hot cars). Also, the natural spring listed on the label could be near a landfill or toxic dump, as was the case in our community. The spring water, reputedly so pristine, might actually be laden with a number of harmful chemicals.

Other Water Hazards: Chlorine in the Swimming Pool

Also potentially harmful are two other members of the fluoride and iodine family: chlorine and bromine. These are lighter and more chemically active than iodine. A chemist would say they are stronger halogens than iodine, meaning that they have a greater affinity for other atoms and bind more strongly with them.

It has been suggested, though not yet scientifically proven, that one way these other halogens interfere with iodine metabolism in the thyroid is by replacing the more weakly bound iodide with a more strongly bound bromide, chloride, or fluoride ion. This might occur if the enzyme forming the molecule was not discriminating enough to tell the difference. The enzyme might be incompetent because of a genetic problem in people who have a tendency for autoimmune thyroiditis.

In her attempt to stay in shape, one of our clients, Judy, started swimming at the local high school pool. The adult swim time was early in the morning, before work, and she thought swimming would be a wonderful addition to her overall health program. After doing a leisurely twenty laps, she would continue with her day. After a couple of weeks of this regimen, she complained: "You know, I feel like I'm losing my marbles lately. I'm feeling all muddled, like I have cotton wool for brains."

When no particular physiological cause for this downturn in cognitive function could be determined, we asked Judy if there had been anything different in her life these last few weeks. "No," she replied. "I keep a very structured program for maintaining my health." When pressed on the issue, however, she remembered, "Oh, yes—I've been swimming these last couple of weeks. This is a change, but one that I thought would help."

As it turned out, the change was not for the better at all. The high level of chlorine in the community pool had begun to adversely affect Judy's delicate thyroid balance. When she stopped the constant added chlorine exposure, her symptoms returned to normal.

There are methods for reducing the amount of chlorine in your personal home pool and/or hot tub. Talk to environmentally friendly pool suppliers who know how, and perhaps consider installing an ozone filter to significantly decrease the chlorine exposure.

Finally, be very frugal in your use of bleaching products that contain chlorine (Clorox and other chlorine bleaches). When you must use such substances, try not to inhale the fumes or have the product come in contact with your skin. Your thyroid may be able to function better because of your caution.

Paper or Plastic?

Twenty-five years ago, our friends, Vic and Mary, lived on their parents' ranch. Unlike their parents, however, they scrupulously avoided the use of plastic wrap on their foods. Back then, we thought such behavior was overly cautious, perhaps bordering on the paranoid. Now, after we have learned that hormone-disrupting plasticizers can migrate into cling-wrapped food, we want to publicly acknowledge Vic and Mary's foresight.

One minimal change you could institute would be to decrease your purchase of cling-wrapped fatty foods. Meat and cheese tend to absorb and retain more hormone-disrupting plasticizers than less fatty items such as breads or vegetables.

People who may be prone to low thyroid function may want to avoid supermarket foods wrapped with plasticizers. Tell the store manager of your personal boycott, and the rationale, in hopes that fewer people will be unknowingly affected. Be sure to remove the supermarket cling wrap as soon as you can, and instead keep your food in cellophane or Glad polypropylene wrap, which does not contain plasticizers.

In 1997, researchers at the FDA discovered that baby bottles made from polycarbonate plastic released bisphenol-A into the bottle contents during heating. This chemical is a plasticizer and a suspected hormone disruptor. Other chemicals may also be released from the bottles. A sensible step might be to go back to using glass. The Evenflow Company now offers tempered glass bottles. Many people still prefer plastic, but they use polyethylene and polypropylene instead of the polycarbonate plastic mentioned above, so as to avoid the plasticizers. Regardless of which type you use, it might still be best not to heat the formula in the plastic itself or to store it there for very long.

Similarly toxic types of plastic are used in toys and toy packaging. Not only baby bottles but also teething rings are made of plastic. It disturbs us that the most vulnerable members of our society eat and drink from containers that may have hormone-disrupting and immune-sensitizing potential. We wonder how it is possible that so many people are unaware of the damage these can inflict on our precious youth.

Heat is also a factor in microwaving food for babies and adults alike. For the reasons mentioned above, it makes the most sense to use glass or ceramic containers in microwave ovens. Even plastic designed for microwave use may contain plasticizers that can leach into the food during the heating process.

If You Can Smell Chemicals, Don't Breathe the Air

Here are some easy measures you can take to improve the air quality in your private living space. Wash the bedding weekly at high temperatures to eliminate dust mites. Have your heating and air conditioning system cleaned and inspected regularly; replace filters every two to three months. Empty and clean the water trays in dehumidifiers, refrigerators, and air conditioners on a regular basis.

Wherever possible, replace carpets with tile, wood, or vinyl floors. Designate your sleeping rooms as more nontoxic and allergy free than the rest of your home. Consider using a Hepa portable air filter in your bedroom. These are now available at any department store. Karilee also keeps a small one in her office.

Autoimmune sufferers should do their best to avoid cigarette smoke, fabric stores (because of airborne particulate matter from the cut edges of material, and the chemicals used in sizing), radiator shops, and newly carpeted or painted rooms. Ants and fleas in the home can be handled quite effectively by nontoxic means. Some companies are now specializing in nontoxic pest control, often using heat or boric acid.

Even closed-air buildings should not escape scrutiny: many people suffer from "sick building syndrome." If you consistently feel worse in a particular building, relocate if that is possible, or buy an air filter for your particular office space. Use hypoallergenic toiletries and scents and less toxic household cleaning products.

Understand the warning hierarchy of labels. "Caution" is the mildest level of concern. "Warning" is stronger, and "Danger" is the most extreme. Make it your business to avoid any products that say "Extra Strength," and instead, choose the ones called "All Purpose," which are generally less toxic.

As for specific alternatives to chemical products, consider the following. Baking soda can be used as a scouring powder instead of chlorine cleansers. Vinegar, in a 50–50 mix with water, makes an excellent all-purpose household cleaner (this is what we use in our home). Club soda, likewise, can be useful in a similar way. It doesn't have to be fizzy; it's the alkaline pH that gives it cleaning power. Another handy safe laundry substitute is borax powder, which can replace some or all of the chemical laundry detergent. Health food stores sell many alternative products that in addition to being safe for use are biodegradable.

Be especially cautious with oven cleaners, drain cleaners, and toilet bowl cleaners. These are best avoided because of the strong chemicals they contain. Instead, you could spray water in the oven, sprinkle bicarbonate of soda over the water, which may help dissolve the heavier buildup, if left on for thirty minutes. You can then use steel wool, with additional water, to remove stubborn stains. Wipe clean with sponge, rags, or paper towels. Instead of using caustic drain cleaners, exercise the preventive measure of putting strainers or traps on your drains, and do what you can to avoid having grease in the sinks. Use toilet bowl cleaners with plant-based surfactants available from health food stores. Consider whether you really need the "super shower scrubbers" with toxic chemicals. For more information, consult the websites, books, and organizations in the Further Reading and Resources sections.

Other Controllable Triggers

If you are already diagnosed with another autoimmune condition, such as diabetes or rheumatoid arthritis, optimal control of this other autoimmune condition will help reduce the autoimmune pressure on your thyroid. Likewise, it might help reduce the autoimmune pressure on your thyroid to avoid possible emotional triggers such as scary movies or particularly noxious people or situations.

On a number of occasions, we had to advise immune-compromised patients to avoid stressful family gatherings in order to preserve what little strength they had. We have had to encourage patients to seek other specialists to work with, when their doctors were acting particularly unsupportive or judgmental.

Exercise great caution regarding exposure to X rays or other possible radiation sources. Some autoimmune thyroid patients believe their symptoms were triggered by X-ray exposure. For an excellent discussion on this topic, see Mary Shomon's book listed in Further Reading.

Inhalant Allergies

For people with environmental allergies, such as to pollen, dust, and mold, you might consider desensitization (a whole body immune system treatment) rather than simply take antihistamines (a symptom reliever). The desensitization process can go a long way toward lowering the overall pressure on your immune system. It involves having some testing done by an allergist and a subsequent regimen of injections or sublingual drops. The extra time and expense for this desensitization might be worth your while in the long run.

The result of certain types of allergy desensitization is an increase in the T-suppressor cells, which, as we have seen, may help reduce the autoimmune response. Other attention to your allergies can help an out-of-balance immune system in similar ways.

Food Allergies

For people who have specific food allergies, the ones they know about are merely the tip of a huge iceberg. Blood tests or skin tests are available to detect other allergenic foods. You can then begin to either avoid or rotate those offenders. This technique is called a rotation-elimination diet, where you avoid the most serious allergens completely and rotate the others, eating them only once every three or four days. For people who appear to be allergic to many common foods, safer bets include lamb, rabbit, fish, potatoes, parsnips, rhubarb, carrots, lettuce, and celery.

One particular, very common food item has a "sticky," sensitizing protein molecule that challenges many people's immune system. It is wheat. Actually, we mean the glutinous, protein component of the wheat, which is also found in oats and rye. The amount of gluten in other grains such as rice, corn, millet, and buckwheat is fairly small.

For many people, gluten intake is a source of continued immune system sensitivity and one that for severe autoimmune low thyroid sufferers is best reduced. (People who are not gluten sensitive need not be concerned with this discussion.) The simplest way to know for sure if you are sensitive to gluten is to take a blood or stool test. The most definitive evaluation for gluten sensitivity is a biopsy done through an endoscopy tube, fed into the small intestine.

It is unclear what makes the gluten molecule so sensitizing to the immune system. It is, after all, the very substance in bread dough that traps gas inside and allows the unbaked bread to rise.

Whatever the cause of gluten intolerance, this problem is more widespread than most people know or than doctors acknowledge. Maybe it's because many people eat gluten-containing products at least three times a day. In the United States, many of us consume glutinous products five or six times each day, whether in major meals (bread and pasta) or in wheat-based snack foods (pretzels, cupcakes, cookies, and crackers).

In certain people, gluten causes from very mild to very severe disruption of the intestinal mucosa. The most severe form of this is called celiac disease, or sprue, also known as severe gluten intolerance. The gliadin portion of the wheat protein acts as an antigen (a molecule that combines with a sensitive person's antibodies) that damages the intestinal cells. In addition to this severe form, there is a whole spectrum of varieties of gluten sensitivity that disrupt the intestine to a lesser degree.

Other foods trigger allergies in a great number of people. Pay special attention to how you feel after eating sugar or dairy products. This latter category is especially sensitizing, perhaps because we are exposed to cow's milk at such an early age and consume it so many times a day well into adult life. The allergic component, the casein protein molecule, has nothing to do with how much or little lactose or fat is in the product we consume.

The intestinal disruption of food allergy often causes malabsorption of needed nutrients. It can also result in absorption of larger food molecules before they are fully broken down. The immune system recognizes these molecules not as a simple carbohydrate or simple fatty acid, but as bits of barley, pork, or asparagus. In other words, they are seen as foreign, causing further immune response. The disorder is popularly known as "leaky gut" syndrome.

This process, called macromolecular absorption, is believed to cause a reasonable degree of additional immune difficulty in certain individuals. When the immune system is already on hyperalert, as is the case with low thyroid sufferers, the disruption can be more severe and debilitating.

If you have known autoimmune problems without known food allergy, be on the lookout for possible food-related symptoms. Many people find that they feel worse after eating certain foods. Some people notice tiredness, dizziness, or a "fuzzy-headed" feeling, in addition to a thick-tongued sensation (not being able to speak or think as clearly). Our suggestion is to listen to your body's wisdom and avoid any foods that cause you to feel in any way uncomfortable. You can also be tested for food allergies, either by blood or skin testing.

One strategy is to eat more hypoallergenic foods, such as brown rice and potatoes in place of the more frequently allergenic wheat starches. Another solution would be to go on a food rotation schedule, eating wheat only every other day or every third day.

Parasites: Facing the Little Demons

The topic of intestinal parasites has received a great deal of press in recent years. According to some, the coverage is well deserved; according to others, it is far-fetched. The issue certainly merits a closer look. We believe that anyone who seriously wants to lessen his or her autoimmune activity should explore carefully the advice to look for and treat any intestinal parasites that can be found. (Severe conditions cause major digestive upset and diarrhea, and are generally treated in order to free people of their debilitating symptoms. Our present discussion is about treating asymptomatic or mildly symptomatic parasite infection.)

We believe that long-term infection with mild intestinal parasites can result in more than just reduced energy or mild intestinal symptoms. It is our definite sense that parasites can be a trigger for the autoimmune phenomenon in sensitive people. The immune system tries to protect the body from what it perceives as an invader, but the intestinal parasite invader generally evades attack by hiding in the intestinal contents.

The inside of the intestine is not really the internal environment of the body, where the immune system reigns supreme. Instead, the inside of the intestine is just out of reach of the immune system, which must work overtime trying to reach the parasitic enemy. This sets the stage, in susceptible people, for enhanced autoimmune activity.

Testing for gastrointestinal parasites is fairly straightforward. Stool samples (either random, or purged with laxative medicines) are collected and analyzed. The difficulty is that most local laboratories find and identify only severe infections. A mild degree or type of intestinal parasite may not be detected.

Fortunately, however, there are a number of special laboratories that are particularly adept at handling these situations. Some receive specimens from all over the country. For a partial listing, see the Resources section. Once identified, intestinal parasites can be well treated with a wide range of both natural and prescription oral medications. We urge you to consult with a qualified and interested practitioner who can assist you in this process.

Long-Term Benefits of Stress Reduction

Stress does affect your immune function. It is certainly known and accepted in medical circles that severe stress can trigger hyperthyroidism, and perhaps Hashimoto's thyroiditis. The exact causal mechanism for this is not clear, but it is tempting to speculate. (Please see Beyond the Tenth Step for a discussion of how "molecules of emotion" might affect your immune status.)

How to De-Stress Your Immune System

For now, suffice it to say that the effects of stress go beyond those described in Step 7 on the adrenal glands. In addition to "fight or flight" reactions that we may actually feel, there are also subconscious fight or flight reactions experienced by our immune system. When stressed on many fronts at once, the immune system may swing into high gear to "protect" us, but the result may be more autoimmunity than protection.

Consider a busy office worker who arrives on the job to find she has a new supervisor. This supervisor, in an attempt to increase efficiency, makes well-intended changes that unfortunately create a hostile environment in the workplace. If the worker is heavily criticized by the new supervisor, she could become increasingly angry and fearful. If the stressful situation continues, her fight or flight response might escalate to a deeper immune response. If this office worker already has a genetic predisposition to a thyroid problem, it is possible that the extra stress, if not handled properly, could trigger the autoimmune thyroid effect.

So what does it mean to handle extra stress properly? We've all heard about stress-reduction activities. When you are going through difficult situations, this is definitely the time to utilize any stress-reduction training you've had. You could choose meditation, self-hypnosis, or specific relaxation exercises from biofeedback or yoga. It is certainly the time to begin getting some exercise or to increase your exercise program, if you already have one. Ideally, you would initiate such a stress-reduction program before you were in the midst of big changes.

This could also be a good time for increased interactions with friends or some counseling sessions with a professional. Many people have found that biofeedback sessions can be very useful during stressful times. The act of quieting the mind using meditation techniques helps relieve the biochemical difficulties caused by the stress.

Several of these techniques are combined in a process known as imagery, which involves imagining yourself in a relaxing locale. It's like a mental vacation. In addition, you can "see" a positive outcome to a problematic situation, or can mentally envision your world getting better. Some call the process visualization, but we find that people are very diverse in the ways they perceive. We use the term "imagery" instead, as imagination can take many forms, including sensations, smells, and feelings. O. Carl Simonton, M.D., Shakti Gawain, Barbara Dossey, R.N., M.S., Jean Acterberg, Ph.D., Martin Rossman, M.D., and many others have popularized the use of imagery for healing.

How to "Call Off the Dogs"

If you suffer from autoimmune thyroiditis, why not visualize your immune system getting smarter and leaving your thyroid alone? Just imagine it getting the point that its best job will be to protect you from outside invaders such as bacteria and viruses. Picture it leaving your glandular system, especially your thyroid, completely free to do its job, unencumbered.

Here is an imagery exercise about "calling off the dogs" that might be appropriate for an overvigilant immune system.

Picture a household (the body) with an empowered older brother named Thomas (the thyroid). It is Thomas's job to keep the home scene running well. He directs everyone else, telling them how hard to work and how fast everything needs to get done. He himself is generally very smartly dressed. Once, while working very hard, however, he changed into overalls and a workshirt. In doing so, the watchdogs (immune system components) failed to recognize him. En masse, all of the dogs began attacking Thomas, making his life and job impossible.

Now suppose that the head of the household (mind and brain) sees what is happening and commands the dogs to immediate attention. He then gently reminds them that Thomas is a trusted member of the household and tells them to leave Thomas alone. The dogs quickly see the error of their ways and sheepishly retire to their former vigilance for outside invaders. Thomas is now able to recover from the attack, and get back to the smooth execution of his job.

The Inner Vacation

Still another imagery exercise that we recommend is as follows:

Picture yourself calmly relaxing in a friendly, natural setting that you have enjoyed in the past. Realize as you view this beautiful scene that the world can be a lovely place, and that you belong here, along with the trees, the birds, and the rest of creation. The world is a safe, inviting place for you to delight in. You can allow your immune system to relax, to take a vacation.

Things here are fine. You have a sense of divine protection, as if you are being watched over by a higher power, and your own personal inner defenses can relax. You might even verbally or mentally affirm, "I am safe. I feel protected. My body and my immune system are at peace with each other. I am at peace with myself and the world."

The medical field specializing in the mind's effect on immunity is called neuroimmunology. Its practitioners and researchers tell us that the brain is constantly communicating with the immune system and that the immune system constantly provides vital information to the brain. Knowing this, you may want to employ positive imagery exercises on a regular basis. You may also want to consider more advanced forms of self-hypnosis and enhanced affirmation strategies. Our own books on this topic are *Healing with Mind Power* and *Creative Imagery in Nursing* (see Further Reading).

Stress Reduction Through Political Activism

We now want to present a nonmedical remedy for autoimmune thyroid disease. This is not a quick fix but a major investment in your community and in your health. You may recall that Dr. Bandura's research on empowerment shows that people who do something about a problem they are facing fare much better than people who remain silent victims of it.

As members of the human family, we must gather our forces as concerned citizens and reduce the polluting of the air, food, and water. There are just too many unnecessary chemicals affecting our immune function adversely. Your political activism regarding this issue may become an important component of your commitment to honor your body.

One of the very best things that you can do for yourself is to exchange ideas and feelings with other people who are similarly challenged. Because of the often invisible, insidious, yet pervasive and multiple effects of this syndrome, people who suffer from it find tremendous benefit in joining together. If possible, meet in small groups. Internet chat rooms and online discussions allow for useful exchange, as well as providing access to the most recent research data in the field. There are so many sites on the Internet that you cannot go wrong if you start with one search word such as "PCB" and go from there. Be sure to explore government environmental websites.

Become attuned to new findings about PCBs, dioxins, plastics, hormone disruptors, and similar environmental toxins. Read the government reports about these substances and the laws pertaining to them.

Complementary Therapies to Ease Autoimmunity

To help recover your former, active, healthy level of well-being, consider the energizing and healing power of acupuncture. Acupuncture is part of a five-thousand-year-old tradition of tapping the body's natural energy. The potential for you to achieve good results with acupuncture's rebalancing qualities is quite high. Many of our patients have found that acupuncture gently guides and opens the flow of their innate healing energy.

Chiropractic can help restore alignment and balance in a system whose metabolic underpinnings have gone astray. Being more comfortable in one's own body is a good first step to relaxing, which then promotes a free flow of hormones. If you are already using chiropractic care and your adjustments "are not holding," consider being checked for thyroid problems. Our experience has been that when people with undiagnosed or borderline low thyroid are unable to maintain a musculoskeletal adjustment, they improve once their system is regulated by the proper dose of thyroid medication.

Another valuable support in achieving a sense of wholeness is massage and bodywork. There are far too many forms of this hands-on therapy to mention here. In general, however, these sessions involve utilizing the skills of a professionally trained practitioner to loosen the muscles, joints, fascia, and body parts, allowing for increased ease, circulation, blood flow, and relaxation. Be sure to include very gentle massage of the neck, especially the lower front thyroid area.

Some people receive massages weekly, others once a month. It is very helpful to work with a certified massage therapist you trust totally, so you are able to direct your consciousness fully to relaxation. Bodywork helps your metabolism to operate more efficiently, flushing out toxins and utilizing nutrients and innate hormones more readily. Be sure to drink plenty of water after massage, because the treatment tends to release several stored metabolites, which then go into circulation and require increased fluid for their elimination.

Beyond massage, there are a variety of subtle yet powerful non-touching "energetic therapies." While many people enjoy massage, others prefer energy healing work that allows them to keep their clothes on. This method of healing is taught and used extensively in the United States and abroad by registered nurses. It is often preferred by people with extreme levels of bodily discomfort, including deep muscle pains and skin problems, both of which can be a result of thyroid disorders.

In addition to the general relaxation benefits of energy therapies, people often notice a deep sense of connection within themselves. At times, they have emotional releases as part of the therapeutic response, so it is best to work with trained professionals who are competent in the emotional aspects of healing.

Like Cures Like

Our final vote of confidence goes to the gentle practice of homeopathy. Homeopathy works by using tiny doses of natural substances that match the individual's personality or situation. (This is known as Hahnemann's law of similars, or the like-cures-like phenomenon.) For example, it's well known that cutting an onion can cause a person's eyes to water. A person who is not cutting an onion, but whose eyes are uncomfortably watering because of a cold or allergy, can find relief by taking a highly dilute form of onion extract *(Allium cepa)* prepared homeopathically into tiny under-the-tongue pellets. Thus, like cures like.

The homeopathic model is in direct contradistinction to Western medicine, which uses substances that oppose or counteract bodily symptoms, as when blood pressure is high, and the person receives strong chemical pills to lower it. Counteracting a body process is called the allopathic approach.

Unlike herbal medicines, which are taken for weeks or months at a time, homeopathic medicines are taken intermittently. The principle can be very helpful to people with low thyroid. The right remedy can make a fundamental change for the better inside the body. We have seen many patients whose autoimmune activity was dramatically diminished after homeopathic treatment. There are currently no allopathic medicines that can duplicate this feat.

For any who doubt the power of the homeopathic principle, consider this classic example. In 1798, Edward Jenner discovered that a very small amount of cowpox material, scratched into a person's arm, could give that individual lifelong immunity to the devastating and highly contagious smallpox virus. This technique, called vaccination, is an incredibly effective preventive medical tool, one that virtually eliminated a terrible disease from the face of the earth. It has since been adapted to defeat many other killer diseases such as polio, tetanus, diphtheria, measles, mumps, and rabies. Vaccination utilizes the "like cures like" principle. The immune system produces antibodies against the vaccine, which protects the person from future exposure to the disease.

The precise biochemical mechanisms involved in the immunization response are some of the most complex in all of medical biochemistry. They illustrate how a minute amount of exactly the right substance, given one time, can have a long-term, beneficial result. This scenario is the basis of homeopathy, a medical system in use all over the world.

In fact, before 1910, a large percentage of the hospitals in the United States were considered to be homeopathic hospitals. Today, the allopaths far outnumber the homeopaths. Yet, as a reminder, both Philadelphia and San Francisco have Hahnemann hospitals, named after the founder of modern homeopathy. In addition, the British royal family, and many well-to-do English, Canadians, and French, use this form of treatment as their preferred medical system.

There are two basic categories of homeopathic treatment: one for acute illness and one for chronic situations. Homeopathic remedies for acute conditions are low-potency and are available at well-stocked vitamin or health food stores. Some pharmacies are starting to carry a few homeopathics, while Rexall has created its own entire line.

Acute, low-potency remedies are sometimes sold as a group in homeopathic first aid kits. Their use is commonly through self-prescription on the basis of the immediate symptoms. We found them very useful to have around the household, especially when our three children were young.

Homeopathic remedies for serious chronic situations are called "constitutional." They are of much higher potency and are available only by advice and administration of a qualified, well-trained homeopathic practitioner (see Resources).

Final Thoughts

We hope that you consider these suggestions for reducing autoimmunity as an exciting optional step. Use only the ideas that seem particularly relevant to you. Consider these ideas a long "menu" with many choices, rather than as a long prescription of necessary actions. We wish you well on your journey.

For those interested in pursuing even more subtle aspects of thyroid recovery, the next step offers an exploration of the intriguing emotional component and its impact on total wellness.

The Bottom Line

- Certain synthetic chemicals are major autoimmune triggers. Reduce your exposure to these potential metabolic toxins, such as insecticides, hair sprays, artificial fragrances, and harsh chemical cleaners.
- Treat your inhalant or food allergies.
- Diagnose and treat mild intestinal parasites.

- Avoid the halogen elements: fluorine, chlorine, bromine, and iodine. Just as noxious are excessively frightening movies and demoralizing people.
- Use stress reduction and imagery techniques to lessen autoimmune activity.
- Further balance your immune system with bodywork, yoga, acupuncture, or homeopathy.

Reach Optimal Recovery with an Empowered Lifestyle

You are not your habits. You can replace old patterns of self-defeating behavior with new patterns.
—STEPHEN R. COVEY, *The Seven Habits of Highly Effective People*

This step is about habits and behavior patterns that either strengthen or diminish us. These habits are patterned in the brain which, the latest science tells us, is continually in dialogue with our immune system. An immune system that is attacking one's own tissues needs some rebalancing and rebuilding. A healthier immune system can result from improved habits and patterns.

The thyroid-compromised person has many avenues to explore in the journey toward greater health and enjoyment of life. We have described several of the best ways we know to enhance physical health. It is now time to move beyond the physical to the realm we call mental or psychological.

In this step, we begin at the level of the individual, with the conclusion of Karilee's personal story. We then move to the group level explored by several thyroid recovery groups with which we've been involved, and where many aspects of relationship are considered. We have found the group's insights to be so useful to our clients that we've distilled some of the best items into "Thyroid Tips" scattered throughout this section. Then we'll expand our view to the societal level—what it means to be an activated consumer and a politically involved planetary citizen, all for the improvement of health and well-being.

Healing on the Individual Level

We hope you will consider this discussion as a way to make connections between physical illness and the meaning of such an experience. We encourage you to explore this crucial body-mind connection, which has the potential to enhance not only your thyroid function but also your total health.

A key aspect of Karilee's odyssey was coming to terms with her chronic disease: not only learning how to cope but how to excel with the challenge. In Step 1, we saw how, after the birth of her second child, Karilee's quality of life had decreased to the point where she was unable to function. However, there was prior evidence that she was suffering from a major illness.

At age twenty, Karilee had gone to Madrid to study Spanish language and culture. There, she found her health compromised but had no understanding of her symptoms. She had increased difficulty in swallowing. Eventually she could not sleep at night unless, lying on her back, she hyperextended her neck over the end of the bed.

At that point, she acknowledged that something was seriously wrong. She also developed a hoarse and raspy voice and felt generally awful. She went to a hospital, where she remained in a bed for a week, steadily becoming worse. Her only treatment was an ice pack on her throat, with no proper diagnosis. Against medical advice, she checked herself out, returned to the United States, and was admitted to Walter Reed Army Medical Center, where she had trained as a student nurse.

Fortunately, there she was given an accurate diagnosis of Hashimoto's autoimmune thyroiditis. The treatment was thyroxine, a synthetic thyroid hormone. This helped tremendously, though never completely. For several years, she took the pills, and eventually began to question if she still needed them. She gradually weaned herself off with no obvious recurrence of symptoms.

Karilee later learned that this reduction of symptoms was not a true disappearance of the illness, but rather its dormant state. Some endocrinologists refer to this quiet period as the calm of a volcano between eruptions. Indeed, many volcanoes that have been dormant for years erupt again unexpectedly. This is exactly what can happen in autoimmune low thyroid disease.

It was after the birth of her second child that the illness again began to rage. At this stage, Karilee had been a vegetarian for a number of years, had practiced yoga and stress-reduction exercises, and believed that she was in excellent health. The return of her thyroiditis symptoms was baffling and upsetting, because she thought she was in total control of her well-being.

Both Karilee and Richard, although medically trained, were unaware that thyroiditis had a tendency to re-erupt. The symptoms of reawakening thyroiditis can be so subtle that even prior low thyroid sufferers might not recognize their reappearance. Symptoms usually increase in number or severity before a doctor puts it all together and diagnoses an "exacerbation of previously compensated thyroid disease." More often, treatment is delivered in a piecemeal, symptom-relief fashion, and can result in years of chasing individual symptoms with little overall relief.

One reason for Karilee's thyroid re-eruption might have been stress. Before the birth of their second child, Karilee and Richard had relocated from a simplified country existence to a complex and more stressful urban environment. Also, her thyroid problem might have been triggered into increased activity by the commonly seen immune activation which occurs postpartum.

There exists a delicate balance between directing one's health and accepting the body one has. Karilee went through a period of soul-searching, exploring many aspects of her psyche and life, in order to understand why she was once again plagued with this energy-depleting illness. At this point, she resumed taking thyroid medication. In a few months, she felt more balanced, regained some of the energy needed to care for her young children, and slowly recuperated from the exacerbation of thyroiditis.

Karilee had loving and nonjudgmental practitioners with whom she worked, who supported her journey. There were others, however, who believed they were empowering her by suggesting that she had chosen this illness. Karilee rejected that idea, and she urges readers of this book to do the same for themselves. You are not to blame for your illness.

After years of sifting through many philosophies about the relationship between disease ("dis-ease") and wellness, Karilee came to an understanding that each person is given a certain physical and emotional constitution within which to stretch and grow. With this foundation, a person can build as strong and beautiful a body as possible, while gaining an acceptance of one's personal familial inheritance and environmental circumstances. She came to see that the lessons resulting from this personal journey are a major part of each person's spiritual path.

One of her greatest problems, after the birth of her second child, was the onset of regular hormone-induced migraine headaches, in addition to the debilitating symptoms mentioned above. These headaches were relentless, excruciating, and incapacitating. As one who had devoted years of professional energy to learning about health and wellness, Karilee was dismayed by her inability to conquer these disabling headaches. She felt if she could just hit upon the "cause" of her migraines, she could eliminate them through natural treatments.

It was a long, humbling experience. Prior to her trial with Imitrex, a newer pharmaceutical treatment for migraines, she would lie flat on her back in a dark room, ice pack on her head, eyes covered, sometimes for two days at a time. She also experienced regular nausea, a severe complication for a nursing mother.

Over the course of fourteen years, she combined her medical treatment with as many natural healing protocols as she could, including acupuncture, movement therapies, craniosacral work, massage and energy therapies, biofeedback, and guided imagery. She eliminated possible migraine triggers, including foods (chocolate, nuts, ice cream, aged cheeses, wines, beer, and more). She also made every effort to avoid environmental triggers, which can vary greatly from individual to individual (for Karilee, some are fluorescent lights, cigarette smoke, intense heat, molds, yeast, dust, and cats). All of these helped somewhat, but nothing fully removed the pain that visited her bimonthly.

In desperation, she made an appointment with the chief professor of neurology at a nearby medical center. He put her on calcium channel-blockers, preventively, and prescribed Imitrex for the relief of a headache already started. In addition, she began working with a new internist to optimize her thyroid medications. He switched her to the new T-3/T-4 regimen of Synthroid plus Cytomel. Better control of the thyroid situation led to better control of the migraines.

These experiences were very empowering to her, but she still did not feel she had all the answers to what was causing her headaches. As she progressed into more subtle healing approaches, she began to believe that there might be many sophisticated diagnostic tools and techniques yet to be discovered.

For example, although these headaches are called "hormonal migraines," no one really understands how migraines and hormones are connected. Some neurologists believe that migraines have nothing to do with anything patients can control. Other neurologists and pain management experts disagree. They think that a variety of migraine triggers can be successfully avoided once they are discovered by diligent observation.

Karilee now has a very full and relatively pain-free existence. Although her low energy and headaches incapacitated her for so many years that she wondered if she would ever be able to live a "normal" life, she now teaches full time on a tenure track at a major university. Her energy is indistinguishable from that of her colleagues. Her migraines are no longer incapacitating, well controlled through her diligent program of combining good medical therapy with good alternative therapy. Although she still has occasional headaches when she "overdoes it," she feels grateful to have a largely normal existence.

The personal path of wisdom, therefore, is one only you can uncover through open-minded exploration, with the support of your health practitioners. It is a remarkable and heroic journey, one that Karilee wholeheartedly recommends to all seeking a more complete recovery of their health.

Healing on the Group Level

Starting in 1993, after working with hundreds of people (mostly women) challenged by thyroid disease, Karilee decided to hold weekly discussion meetings in her office for people coping with thyroid disorders. She invited a number of the clients she and Richard were seeing to participate in thyroid recovery groups. Information presented here about group members uses assumed names to protect their privacy.

Many people have found it enormously useful to explore the meaning of their disease in this type of safe group setting. The women in these groups could find support for their belief that they don't have to accept feeling terrible much of the time. They could listen to each other's stories, learn and share together, and empower each other.

Hints About Physical Comfort
Eventually, Karilee's project coalesced into several small, highly committed groups of seven to ten women who met biweekly for two or three years. They evolved from telling their stories to search-

ing for answers, first on the physical level; then on the psychological level.

Members took turns doing research and eagerly shared information they had learned from books or other sources, as well as sharing how they felt when they tried the various remedies.

Many participants revealed feelings of being out of control and unable to cope, occasionally experiencing severe depression, fatigue, anxiety, and labile moods (ranging from extremely hyper and anxious to very low and depressed). Around the time of menstruation, many of the women reported feeling "off the wall," with decreased mental capacity, often not able to complete sentences or think clearly. In fact, several reported severe episodic memory loss.

For low episodes, 200–300 milligrams of the herbal medicine St. John's Wort, once daily, was helpful to some. Quite a few participants found they felt healthier when they took extra fiber or digestive enzymes to counteract low thyroid's sluggish bowel symptoms.

Some reported feeling better using memory-enhancing supplements such as ginkgo biloba (40 milligrams three times a day). When they felt increased autoimmune inflammation of the thyroid gland, they often improved with the herb willow bark (two tablets, taken two or three times a day). Some used magnesium tablets (200 milligrams three times a day) to help with occasional palpitations, and valerian root (two or three capsules three times each day, especially at bedtime) to promote calm and relaxation.

Group members experimented together at times, such as when they decided to have a trial period eliminating programmed television from their "activity diet." Most of the women felt better and more energized when not watching television, believing that perhaps its continuous barrage of negativity and violence impacted their health.

Some did research in the library and reported on studies revealing negative effects of television viewing on immune function.

> *Thyroid Tip* Carefully consider all sources of input into your life, and screen out those that may be draining your energy or making you feel worse.

The conclusion the groups generally reached was that anyone embarking on combined physical and psychological thyroid treatment should not be surprised to experience an initial exacerbation of symptoms, prior to stabilizing and fine-tuning. Several group members with longstanding histories required a complete program for achieving optimal health, including nutritional advice, exercise coaching, and psychological counseling.

The Journey of Self-Discovery

The group helped members come to terms with the fact that most people with chronic thyroid problems go through predictable stages, as does anyone when facing a long-term chronic illness. First, one needs to accept having more than a mild imbalance. This process can be complicated because people can find their self-esteem diminished by acknowledging the presence of an illness or disease.

After the initial and sometimes hard-to-overcome reluctance to accept having an illness, the person may experience many feelings. She may want to be taken care of and nurtured, or she may react by pulling back, not being fully open with others who, she believes, can't possibly understand. She may feel angry, betrayed by her body, and confused.

> *Thyroid Tip* Emotions are a normal, healthy response to being diagnosed with any condition, including that of low thyroid, and

most people will benefit from having support for resolution of these issues.

Some never get beyond this stage, but many proceed to acceptance and to a sense of needing to empower themselves and others. An important overriding theme emerged in these groups. All the members were able to identify what seemed to be a similar disorder in their approach to life. They all felt "hypervigilant," guarded against the world and its stressors.

Another commonality they uncovered was that almost everyone in the groups described herself as hypersensitive and feeling like the proverbial "canary in a coal mine." (Long ago, coal miners kept canaries in cages down in the mines because the birds were more sensitive to the deadly but odorless gases that would sometimes escape into a mine shaft. When the canaries died, that signaled the miners to evacuate immediately.)

Modern day "canaries" are people who seem to be more sensitive than others to the hazards of modern life. Their resulting illness can serve as a warning to the population at large, signaling that impending environmental hazards are worsening.

Thyroid Tip Often those with autoimmune thyroid are extremely sensitive people, perhaps reacting more quickly or strongly to an external threat that may eventually affect everyone.

On the other hand, however, they found that their overly watchful immune systems were, at times, protecting them from the wrong things, i.e., they were attacking their own tissues. The groups' decision was that those who are challenged in this particular way need to make better friends with themselves and boost self-esteem.

Thyroid Tip People with autoimmune challenges may be on "hyperalert," and can benefit from rebuilding their defenses into something more healthy and discriminating.

In the groups, members consciously chose to regard the thyroid disease as an experience, a journey about "surrendering" and "opening up to the process." These ideas may be familiar, having originally been described by Dr. Elisabeth Kübler-Ross in her famous book, *On Death and Dying.*

Autoimmunity and Self-Esteem

Participants spent considerable time exploring issues of self-esteem with the body as a metaphor for "self." The body has a natural defense system, alerting us to potential harm. When one has an autoimmune low thyroid, one's body rejects aspects of itself, attacking, in this case, the thyroid gland. This attack proceeds as if the gland were a spy or foreign invader, rather than a valued member of the body's team.

Here was another common thread. Many felt that some "central control" within was rejecting a part of themselves. Where might such rejection originate? As they delved deeper, many discovered that family rejection in early life was one common source.

Thyroid Tip For many people with autoimmune thyroid, benefit may be derived from considering the meaning of "protection" and "rejection" in their lives.

For Suzanne, especially, the pieces of a large blurry puzzle began to take form. She sensed there might be something vitally important for her about the theme of early rejection. One myth had particular meaning for Suzanne. The story "The Mistaken Zygote," from the book *Women Who Run with the Wolves* by Clarissa Pinkola Estes, illustrated how Suzanne felt about her family of origin. In this ethnic folk tale, espousing a common theme in many cultures, a fertilized egg was supposed to be "delivered" to the home of a certain family, but the bird became confused and dropped it elsewhere. The individual grew up with a different family, and was very puzzled and uncomfortable.

Suzanne felt that many of her own characteristics were not consistent with those of her family. She certainly felt as if she didn't fit well into her family of origin, and occasionally fantasized about having been adopted. Suzanne considered that feeling like an outsider in her "clan" could have been a factor in the development or triggering of her autoimmune thyroid tendency.

Thyroid Tip Since the mind and body are intricately interconnected, for optimal recovery one must carefully guard one's thoughts, weeding out those which are immune-disruptive.

Another relevant folk myth is "The Ugly Duckling" by Hans Christian Andersen. In this story the mother duck has one egg that takes too long to hatch. When it finally hatches, the duckling is different, and the other ducks criticize him. He grows up teased, rejected, and feeling unloved. Once mature, he sees his reflection to find that he is now a beautiful swan. No one recognized his true self until this time, and he now comes to be honored and appreciated.

Almost all the group participants described an "ugly duckling" childhood where they didn't feel safe or valued. Some had parents who were verbally abusive and labeled them with derogatory words. A child, vulnerable and reliant on a parent, may learn a variety of coping responses as a result of this kind of treatment. These often include not expressing one's inner feelings or truth, not feeling safe sharing oneself fully in the world, and not knowing how to relate in a healthy manner to others. All such behaviors undermine and attack the self.

Relationships

Since many in the groups were tired so much of the time, they had to learn ways to conserve energy. They agreed on the need to limit "energy suckers," people who manipulated and drained their energies in order to feed their own needs. They had to learn to identify this type of interaction immediately when it occurred.

Here is how they did it. Most of them had such people in their lives: a nosy neighbor, an abusive or ineffectual boss, a child with temper tantrums, a widowed parent with learned helplessness, or a chatty friend with fewer demands and responsibilities. They came to realize that these people behave in parasitic ways unconsciously, not necessarily intending to drain energy from others, but acting compulsively in a way they learned in their early life to get attention. Group members who were energetically deprived, however, could not afford to have energy-suckers feed off them!

Thyroid Tip Certain people may affect your health in ways that are immuno-disruptive.

Once they learned to respect and honor themselves, group members learned how to define boundaries within a loving relationship.

They found themselves redefining their needs and desires, identifying what they would and would not do, what they expected others to do, and how the family would reorganize itself around a democratic pattern rather than an autocratic one. They empowered each other with the strength and courage to set these limits. They learned to find a balance, and to recognize when they lost it.

Perfectionism, Addiction, and Compulsive Behavior

Another rampant destructive behavior that was identified was perfectionism. Members were often afraid to take risks, fearful that they might not do a job perfectly. Dependence versus independence was a struggle. As many psychologists have found, perfectionism is one source of the tendency toward addiction. Many also saw their tendency to assume the role of victim. Most felt a lack within themselves, as if they had a serious defect that could never be corrected, no matter how much they tried to rebuild themselves.

Addiction to work was common, assessed as a desire to escape from life's other challenges by burying themselves in a behavior that had proven successful. These women differed from those who became overly involved, and then became overwhelmed and stymied. Many in the groups were incredibly responsible and followed through with their duties at great personal cost. Sometimes the high price included weight gain, sugar addiction, chronic tiredness, foggy-headedness, food cravings, self-reproach for not expressing anger appropriately, and subsequent lowered self-esteem.

Others may recognize these ideas from twelve-step programs, which also help to support people in moving beyond harmful patterns. The twelve steps encourage people to accept what cannot be changed, to change what they can, and to gain the wisdom to know the difference (which can be the tricky part!).

Many also were compulsively active, wanting to go, go, go constantly. Others identified an overwhelming need to control fully every aspect of their lives. They gradually learned how to release these and other behavior patterns that were not serving their highest good. They were aware that the medical establishment had yet to understand the depth and multidimensionality of their illness. No one felt that her small group had the answers for everyone, but each hoped that the group's explorations might help expand awareness and understanding of this difficult disease.

Group members frequently had a good laugh when listening to each other. When analyzing one woman's patterns, they all could see the same vicious cycle in themselves. Jessica's story was typical. First she wanted her home to be perfect. She vacuumed, dusted, straightened, threw away, repaired and painted the walls, purchased new curtains, washed and ironed them, then hung them while cooking dinner. She watched her children to make certain that they dressed impeccably.

Jessica could tolerate no slouching in any aspect of her life. She joined the PTA and the League of Women Voters, helped lead a Girl Scout troop, and volunteered at the local women's center. She took a course in computers to keep up with technological changes. When her husband returned from work, she always had a balanced meal ready for him. When he finished eating she cleared the table and washed the dishes. And she just couldn't answer the constant nagging question "Why am I so tired?"

Discussion of Jessica's situation led the group participants to set a goal of taking back their power. Many of them felt they had long been overly controlled through male dominance, accepting their lifestyle as normal. The roles that they played were reexamined through the lens of a more modern family structure where all members contribute to its smooth maintenance.

Thyroid Tip Setting boundaries and avoiding compulsive behaviors might be very significant ways to conserve energy when compromised.

Women shared unhealthy coping patterns they had developed, including other compulsive behaviors. One pattern was to overindulge, to do something (eat, spend, talk) compulsively, in an attempt to feel better, often justifying the behaviors by saying, "I deserve this," or "I need this in order to cope." In order to achieve a more positive sense of balance, these women learned to ask, "What do I really need?" rather than acting in a driven manner.

They slowed down their behavior, identified the difference between acting and reacting, and learned to identify triggers to their reactive behavior. They began to see that they were pushing to accomplish, to do, to create, to express, in order to avoid facing their own unpleasant feelings, including the feeling of exhaustion, deep inside.

Carla articulated a fascinating insight. "I now like to think of my immune system as run by a kindly and wise diplomat, one who prefers to have no enemies, who sees that everything has its right place and function. My healthy immune system allows for harmonious interactions all around. It has to be neutral, seeing worth and value in everything. If it gets out of balance, there may be hateful judgment and excessive overvigilance, leading to battles and war. Of course, its rightful job is to mobilize forces appropriately, to attack if necessary, to weed out enemies. But now I try to instruct it to do its rightful job, only when absolutely necessary, only after gentle diplomacy has been fully explored."

Thyroid Tip Take some time to consider a positive mental image for your immune system that helps you to make the best decisions for your health.

Conflict—Internal and External

Insights frequently led to more insights—in oneself or in others. Suzanne noted that she had been eating everything in sight for months and had thought it might just be an attempt to boost her energy. After hearing Mary, however, she began to think she might be "stuffing" the rage she felt toward her husband, who continually belittled her.

Carla suggested that members could call upon the "internal diplomat" of the immune system as a way to correct their compulsions when they noticed themselves acting in this manner. Some groups did imagery exercises and one, led by Carla, envisioned their "inner diplomat" telling their immune systems to act wisely and judiciously.

Their new goal was to practice "not reacting," and to recognize an alarm response sooner. They did this first by not allowing themselves to become overtired, which is a major stressor for people with these conditions. They also sought to prevent the situations that made them feel out of control, that otherwise might escalate into a rage response. They learned to monitor themselves more carefully, to pay attention to subtle cues that informed them when their immune system was going on red alert.

Some participants tended to direct anger outward, blaming and criticizing those around them. Others directed the rage inward, with resultant lowered self-esteem and depression. The members unanimously agreed that both methods were equally ineffectual and damaging. They made a commitment to write some of their deepest feelings in a journal to help release them and to strive for earlier intervention (talking out their concerns) before they became totally upset.

Some, especially those with young children, even found benefit from beating pillows in their rooms, and screaming into pillows to avoid expressing their rage inappropriately. Anger management, and clear expression of inner emotions, was a goal they all agreed on. Many psychologists recommend these safe-setting emotional discharge sessions as a way to release anger without causing it to escalate in oneself or others.

Thyroid Tip Anger management can be a key to stabilizing the thyroid and improving overall health.

The head and heart can often be at odds, as many of us find in our daily lives. However, thyroid-compromised individuals cannot afford to have needless battles. They must choose their battles wisely and expend energy cautiously and appropriately.

Their Mothers' Daughters

A number of women expressed that they experienced conflict, often anguish, when interacting with their mothers. Many had to cope in early life with the challenge of an emotionally immature mother and felt they had been put in a position where they had to "raise" their mothers. Metaphorically, they "shouldered" the weight of their responsibility.

They considered the possibility that the body mirrored some inner aspects of their lives. One woman commented that her mother always called her a "pain in the neck." She wondered if that could have anything to do with her ongoing thyroid dilemmas.

Others had mothers who were frequently out of control (possibly also due to thyroid disease). Several had mothers who behaved like a jealous competitor if the daughter received positive attention from the father.

Thyroid Tip Many women with autoimmune low thyroid seem to benefit from exploring and improving their relationship with their mothers.

Wendy told the story of how her mother took her to the shopping center to buy her first lipstick when she was twelve years old. When Wendy didn't like her mother's choice of colors, her mother became enraged, and publicly beat her, screaming, "I'm going to beat those breasts back into your chest." This horrifying, yet revealing statement is obviously from a mother who was having a lot of unresolved feelings about her daughter's budding femininity, perhaps related to her own waning attractiveness.

Group members noticed that when they improved their lives and circumstances, their mothers also seemed better. In order to improve, they had to detach, at times, from their mothers. Some visualized their mothers in a protective bubble to help themselves separate, grow, and thrive. Their combination of low energy and extreme sensitivity made this detachment crucial.

Thyroid Tip Learning to detach from the negative behavior of family members can be immune-enhancing at times.

Carla found that if she saw her mother for a day and a half, no longer, whenever the mother came to visit, things worked out well. After that amount of time, the mother would become more and more "comfortable," reverting to old, unconscious patterns and behaviors. So Carla learned to limit her mother's visits, despite her mother's protests. Mother and daughter then had a more positive, healthy relationship.

Thyroid Tip Clear communication can be immune-enhancing.

A woman's relationship with her mother can be so close that it can be very difficult to find a healthy balance. While many daughters wish to reject the aspects of themselves that are like their mothers, we have to admit our mothers are in our genes. And, for all the challenges, we love them and wish them well.

Personal Momentum

People with low thyroid must focus on taking tiny steps and evaluating their progress over the long haul, rather than striving for huge progress in a hurry. They must learn to take things one day at a time, in order to avoid being overwhelmed. In addition, they must learn to honor their improvements, no matter how small.

Julie said, "I know I'm doing well when I have more good days than bad days. To me, after a lifelong battle with energy depletion, this is progress!" For Carla, being able to take a walk without feeling depleted was a "good day." If Suzanne could have a conversation with her sister without becoming angry, this constituted a step forward.

Thyroid Tip People with low thyroid need to honor their own pace and abilities on a day-to-day basis, without judgment or comparison.

For Mary, just taking thyroid medication was a big step in the right direction. She had resisted taking medication for many months, hoping that she could make other changes that would boost her energy. When nothing else gave her the sense of well-being she was looking for, she implemented a regimen of thyroid medication, taking a very small dose. Within days, she began to feel more like her old self. For her, this was the next step. For many, taking thyroid medication can be the difference between waking with joy or dread.

As Wendy observed, "Sometimes I feel as if my whole life is my illness." Her challenge was to be responsive to her health problems, without becoming obsessed with them. Another woman related: "I would not have made it through the last twelve to fifteen years without having daily meetings with my husband, sharing how I felt and what I needed. He understands because he also has health problems."

Group Support of Individual Differences

Humans have a tendency to compare themselves to others. Unfortunately, the competitive feeling this arouses in some people leaves them feeling less than whole. A severely negative self-assessment can leave some individuals feeling despondent. For that reason, group members were discouraged from comparing their progress or severity of symptoms. Some did compare their own progress: good days versus bad days, or what they could do now versus what they could or couldn't do last week. This proved a problem at times, since energy levels can fluctuate.

Thyroid Tip "Comparison can be a cancer of the spirit" (attributed to Gerald Jampolsky, M.D., in his lectures).

Group members needed to be willing to explore different approaches, honoring their feelings as a guide to what made sense for them, right in that moment. They learned to view events in their lives as lessons, rather than as successes or failures. Through their group interactions, many learned to be kinder to themselves and to be guided by their inner voice.

Each group learned to acknowledge and honor individual forms of emotional expression. One participant initially reported, "I either blow it all out, or else I check out." This referred to her pattern of either releasing rage or closing down and withdrawing in difficult situations.

After several months of heart-centered group experiences, she finally said: "I used to totally disconnect from whatever was upsetting. Now I can hang in there and make better choices about each situation, choices that empower everyone. It's all about setting boundaries, and about what I do with my emotions."

Out of a growing appreciation for the uniqueness of each individual, group members then spent time helping each other to identify their history, attitudes, beliefs, and genetic inheritance, all integral components of individuality. This helped them decipher the messages the body was providing, in order to move toward a higher level of health and well-being.

Thyroid Tip At times, recovery can be enhanced by unlearning poor habits and replacing them with kind and respectful self-care.

Healing on the Societal Level

There is a concept known as "the hundredth monkey." This refers to the observations of a Japanese primate specialist who noticed that once a critical mass of exposure to a new idea occurs, it spreads rapidly in ways that science cannot explain.

As health care providers, we think that awareness of the thyroid epidemic is so vitally important to our society that it must be disseminated to the populace through a grass-roots process. Not only will this information help our society at large, but, in addition, health activism is part of the rebuilding and restoration of your personal defense system into something more healthy and discriminating.

Finding One's Voice

In *The Thyroid Solution,* Baylor Medical Center endocrinologist Ridha Arem wrote about the psychological aspects of low thyroid. He contends that there are unique behaviors exhibited by low thyroid patients due to its multiple effects on the body and mind. Healing this disease, for some, means putting enough value on themselves to speak their truth and defend it.

A person with heart disease must learn to honor the call of the heart (love, forgiveness, rest, and peace). People with thyroid disease must learn to honor their voice. Group members asked themselves, "What stops us from speaking our truth?" They found that it was often hard to believe that what they had to say was worthwhile. In the group setting, they gradually learned that others did indeed want to hear from them.

In Eastern tradition, the throat is the fifth major energy center (see Beyond the Tenth Step), relating to communications and self-expression. The thyroid gland itself is close to the voice box (larynx). Inflammation of the gland often affects both speech and swallowing. The feeling of "choking up" when we are afraid to speak out involves a tightening of the muscles in the throat, which, if habitual, can result in decreased blood and lymph flow to the thyroid gland.

Evelyn's Story: One Example of Empowered Attitude

Evelyn, an early group member, had a particularly compelling story to share. "It started with my noticing some unusual symptoms, including swollen feet, difficulty adjusting to temperature changes, and profound fatigue. This was the beginning of my hypothyroid time. It got so bad I couldn't carry groceries from my car to the kitchen.

"I remember breaking down and crying one afternoon. Here I was, a very successful businesswoman, and I had no energy to do a task that seemed so simple. This severe hypothyroid experience, which I had for several months, was the most difficult time of my life. I felt like an invalid. I now feel deeply for those who have the condition of low thyroid all the time.

"I didn't want to go on living this way, so I made a decision that I would in fact heal myself. My first step was to obtain good medical care from an understanding practitioner regarding this new situation in my life. My next step was to read every book I could find that described my condition, its medications, and their effects. I did everything I could to learn more about my condition (I continue to be reluctant to call it a 'disease'). I began to focus on my life, my mind, and my circumstances, to discover what might have possibly generated this condition in me.

"I have a tremendous sense of my own power, and I have great belief in the mind's ability to heal. I read a book called *Remarkable Recovery* [see Further Reading], because I wanted evidence that it was possible for me to cure my condition. I decided that if people could cure terminal cancer and brain tumors, I could heal my thyroid condition, and change whatever it was that created it.

"Then I took a serious look at my life. It was very out of balance. I had been a workaholic, with my life so busy and requiring so much energy that my thyroid might have burned out from all these demands.

"For the purpose of deeper healing, I dramatically altered my professional life. Now I work about three and a half days per week instead of seven full days a week. My thyroid condition was a blessing in disguise. It was responsible for, and contributed to, my now living a more balanced life.

"I also looked at circumstances that might have been additional triggers, besides my work life. I read that thyroid flareups often occur after a major loss, such as losing a job or relationship. My mother had died recently, and a very significant romantic relationship had ended unexpectedly. I therefore knew I had to make some adjustments in my spiritual and psychological life. I began to get involved with counseling and participating in meditation and spiritual retreats. To this day, I continue to do these things.

"This is a beautiful example of how following the clues in my life has enabled me to transcend certain barriers, and move into my power. I have a shelf of books on hormone balance. I was able to find an endocrinologist who trusts me, works with me when I want to change my medications, and allows me to have blood tests when I feel they are necessary. He says I know more about this condition than he does!

"Thus, I recommend that you find a physician who will be your partner, with mutual respect and trust. Everything teaches us, and I believe in honoring the body as teacher."

Evelyn now shares her story with anyone who will listen. She writes books and lectures across the country. Her constant goal seems to be to change health care for the better and upgrade society.

Consumer Empowerment

The realizations of the thyroid recovery group members occurred over several years of slow and careful exploration. Karilee hopes that you "try on" whatever fits, and make use of it where appropriate. Simply ignore or discard whatever doesn't seem meaningful to you.

Karilee obviously believes in the body-mind-spirit approach to health, as well as the doctor-nurse-patient (team) approach. This philosophy teaches that the best solutions for a chronic condition like autoimmune low thyroid result from the joining of minds and hearts, sharing hope and knowledge freely for the betterment of all.

According to Florence Nightingale, founder of modern nursing, in her famous book, *Notes on Nursing* (see Further Reading), "Nature alone cures . . . and what nursing has to do is to put the patient in the best condition for nature to act upon him." This line of thinking led Nightingale to the societal challenge of revamping the British health administration. More of her kind of political activism is needed today for our current thyroid epidemic. Speaking out on the politics of health care was a consistent group recommendation.

The Journey Home

Although the initial focus in the thyroid recovery groups was to explore symptom reduction, its emphasis evolved into a focus on medical politics and societal healing. The idea of injecting enthusiasm into the process, rather than fear or gloom, created a shift in the way the groups functioned. Participants became tired of talking about problems and began to focus more on solutions, on what was working, and on how empowered they felt when they were actively involved in their health process, generally feeling more balance in their lives.

Most participants ended up seeing their illness as a teacher, rather than as a plague. Describing it with more neutral terminology, they felt less victimized and more in control, which in itself led to a greater sense of autonomy and enjoyment of life.

Do not let anyone tell you how you feel, what you think, or what you believe. If you had overbearing parents or teachers in early years, you may have developed a pattern of allowing others to define you and your immune balance. Those currently in control of your destiny may be politicians, health bureaucrats, or insurance company employees. As health professionals, we strongly advise that you consider speaking out, individually and collectively, to these groups to improve your own health and quality of life.

Our work with thousands of people has taught us that each person's healing is an intimate process, one in which we are deeply honored to participate. We do not presume to heal people, but we can be with them as they do the deep healing work of defining and refining themselves, just as the group members did.

Caroline had been a busy political activist before her thyroid system became depleted. She had to adjust to doing much less and cried the day she said she could no longer participate in these activities, which were so important to her. After sharing her despair, she explored her options enough to realize that with the donation of an old computer from one of the group members, she would be able to continue her campaigning via email.

Do not allow your voice to remain silent. Know that one voice can make a difference. Look back to 1950, when a lone canary, by the name of Rachel Carson, sang a sad song, telling us of the potentially devastating effects of pollution in the environment. Interestingly, at the time Rachel Carson had breast cancer.

Her passionate book, *Silent Spring* (see Further Reading), is a classic today, an inspiration for current books that sing in harmony with her warning from long ago. Speak out, as part of your healing journey. Pay attention to your body, your feelings, and the data, and help your community to make the best decisions for the largest number of people.

Many of the thyroid group members are continuing their journey together. As their own healers, they do yoga, aerobic exercise, stress-reduction, and imagery. They take natural substances to augment and balance their chemical medicine. They regulate their activities according to the messages they get from their bodies. They use their symptoms as barometers for how they live their daily lives.

These various group members are taking large steps toward accepting their power as healers of themselves and the planet. Karilee encourages others with low thyroid to find similar meaning and support on their journey toward health and wholeness.

The Bottom Line

- Consider becoming involved with a support group that can help you explore options and feel connected throughout your recovery process.

- Pick supportive, nonjudgmental practitioners to assist in your health recovery efforts.
- With an empowered attitude, you can rebuild your defenses into something more healthy and discriminating.
- Health is not a goal or destination, but is an ongoing process. Enjoy the trip, and let your voice be heard.

How to Tap the Source of Boundless Energy

The most beautiful thing we can ever experience is the mysterious. It is the true source of all art and science—explore the unknown boldly.

—ALBERT EINSTEIN, *What I Believe*

We hope you consider this book your invitation to a healthier and more robust and energetic life. It is our heartfelt belief that optimizing thyroid function is an excellent place to start.

Even if you boost your metabolism into normal range using the methods presented in our ten steps, this is only the beginning of a total vitality program. Balancing your energy is a process that involves an ongoing commitment to greater health and well-being.

All of us have at our disposal far more healing energy than we ordinarily realize or use. Learning to liberate this huge reservoir of power is one of life's greatest challenges. Now that you've seen how to optimize your energy hormones, you can combine this improvement with certain other health activities to profoundly improve your over-all vitality.

We now offer some remarkably effective suggestions, but only for those who wish to go beyond the commonly accepted approaches. To have obtained your diagnosis, you may have needed to go beyond the standard diagnostic criteria. Whether you now wish to go well beyond the standard treatment criteria is purely a matter of personal choice.

Some people are most comfortable with their total thyroid pro-gram consisting of one Synthroid pill each morning. Others prefer a more complex program that might also include Cytomel, nutritional supplements, immune modulation, and psychological awareness. Perhaps you will want even more.

There is no one best thyroid program for everyone. The purpose of this book has been to help you utilize current science in developing an individualized program for yourself. If you are one of those open-minded people who wants to experiment with additional information beyond present-day medical science, then please read on. We hope you enjoy entertaining the possibility of power that transcends cur-rent scientific understanding.

An Expanded View of Health

To take full advantage of this power, we need to expand our concept of health. An impressive amount of research data confirms the value of adopting a holistic and multidimensional paradigm.

The goal of modern medicine has been geared toward curing, generally measured as a removal of symptoms. Health providers are divided, however, on how best to heal. Physicians are concerned with outcomes, while nurses are involved more with process. As a doctor-nurse team, we have seen patients "cured" again and again. The symptoms are assuaged, but the recidivism rate is high. Some of the new symptoms are even more serious than the initial presenting ones. Have we helped those patients to heal?

Health is a dynamic process, not a state of being. The word "health" has as part of its meaning "hale, hearty, whole, holy." Healing is a process that implies "making whole." We have seen many instances of patients being "cured," yet not achieving health: a sense of being whole.

In order to heal, one must do more than eliminate symptoms; one must address the root cause of the symptoms. A patient who is healed does not return again and again, with the same or different symptoms. He or she is able to break free of this unhealthy cycle.

In this section, we will explore how modern health providers can augment their science with age-old approaches to true healing. Holistic practitioners can serve as a bridge between various healing models, allowing for both conventional and alternative approaches to be integrated and applied. They can provide skills, tools, information, and support that can help consumers empower themselves to make some profoundly useful changes. We hope that each of the following ideas can serve as a stepping stone for your journey toward total vitality.

A Growing Appreciation for the Body-Mind

In the 1970s, groundbreaking body-mind research was done at the National Institutes of Health. While exploring the body's chemical messengers and their receptor sites, Candace Pert, Ph.D., made a discovery that not only defined her career as a scientist but also changed the way scientists view the human organism.

The chemical messengers she studied most were peptide neurotransmitters and their receptors. Peptides are molecules made from chains of amino acids. These chains are essential to the body's maintenance and growth. Neurotransmitters are chemicals that are active at the synapse connection between nerve cells. Receptors are sites on cells that function as sensing stations, where chemical messengers have their effect.

The peptide messenger attaches to the receptor, creating a disturbance, which "tickles" the receptor molecule into rearranging itself, changing its shape until information enters the cell. This lock and key process is known as binding. In her book, Pert refers to this as sex on the molecular level (see Further Reading).

Pert mapped the distribution of receptors in the brain and found that the limbic system, considered to be the seat of emotions, contained the largest percentage of neuropeptide receptors. Over the course of many years of diligent research, she found that many of the peptides active in the brain are actually manufactured and released into the bloodstream by body organs other than the brain.

In other words, the origin of the brain's emotions is spread out all over the body. The mind, therefore, is all over the body as well. In fact, the body is the subconscious mind.

Pert's work helps us to comprehend the interconnectedness between mind and body, and between emotions and immunity. She coined the term "molecules of emotion" to describe the interaction of peptides and receptors involved in the expression of human feelings.

This information helps us to comprehend the many intricate chemical connections that define each person. The thyroid is merely one gland in a vast glandular network, creating chemicals that flow throughout the body, interacting with chemicals from various other organs, producing more complex chemicals that go back and forth between brain and body, establishing who we are and how we function.

It is now clearer than ever before that the immune system is not an autonomous self-regulating entity but instead is involved with the brain and the mind in a constant conversation. This discovery represents an enormous and previously unrecognized body-mind intelligence that we can use to keep ourselves healthy.

As modern medicine begins to put the pieces of this grand puzzle together, we have more opportunity to heal, to become whole, and to actualize our unique and complete potential as humans. In learning to keep ourselves well, we can inspire healthier attitudes in those around us. We can thus use this knowledge and understanding to create a more viable and sustainable planet, which can nourish us all.

A Model for Self-Actualization

In addition to working directly with the physiology of body-mind, healing professionals have renewed interest in the topic of subtle body energies. If indeed the mind is all over the body, what might be its overall organizing structure? Moreover, how might one use knowledge of such organization for improving health and vitality?

Basic Energy Field Theory

For thousands of years, practitioners of Eastern religions have described an enveloping energy field surrounding the physical body. According to energy field theory, humans are more than simply a body, with electrical and chemical activity occurring inside. Instead, what we call the body is simply the densest part of the human energy field. Extending beyond the physical body are the more subtle aspects of the person.

It might help to envision this energy field as a template or framework upon which the human form is built. The easiest way to think about it is to picture architectural drawings. These two-dimensional representations determine how a three-dimensional building will eventually look. The human energy field is like these architectural drawings: spirit is the blueprint, mind is the builder, and body is the result.

For those who doubt the existence of the human energy field, consider these medical tests: the electrocardiogram (EKG), the electroencephalogram (EEG), and the new magnetoencephalogram (MEG). These well-documented evaluations are merely measurements of three different types of electrochemical waves emanating from a human being. Just a few generations ago, their existence would have been the subject of educated guesses and speculation. In a few more generations, today's educated speculation about subtle energy fields may well become tomorrow's commonplace scientific measurement. In fact, there are scientists in southern California and southern Japan currently developing instrumentation to measure the biofield.

Since earliest recorded human history, there have been people who did not require electrical instruments for this purpose. They seemed to possess highly attuned perceptive skills and were known as the village "seers" or healers. Sensitive individuals are able to "read" another person's subtle energies. Some see the energy field as an aura of light and color emanating from the body. This aura may have been suggested by Byzantine and pre-Renaissance artists, who often depicted Jesus and Christian mystics with a halo around their heads.

The aura or halo of energy around a person can now be understood as a field of information about that person, existing in various layers, progressing from the denser physical layer to the less dense emotional layer, and to the even less dense mental and spiritual layers. These layers are overlapping and interconnected. This concept of interconnecting energy layers is consistent with the scheme of nursing theorist, Dr. Martha Rogers, who taught that humans are multidimensional energy fields—irreducible, unitary, and whole.

Healers with highly developed intuitive skills can read the information surrounding the body, assisting people in understanding their life challenges more completely. Health care consumers can learn to read their own internal messages as well.

The Organizational Hierarchy

To establish a framework for the concept of energetic healing, we've included a diagram demonstrating the correlation between a modern Western model familiar to many—Maslow's Hierarchy of Needs, and the ancient yogic system of energy centers or chakras.

The founder of humanist psychology, Abraham Maslow, proposed a now widely accepted model that conveys a hierarchy of human need. Maslow's intensive search for a comprehensive theory of human behavior led him to develop a model that synthesized art and science, incorporating poetry, philosophy, religion, art, values, and scientific principle.

According to Maslow's model, people must first tend to basic physical needs (air, water, food, safety, security, physical comfort) prior to moving up the ladder to meet intermediate goals (acceptance, approval, recognition). From there, they can move on to loftier goals (self-fulfillment, realization of one's potential). Since Maslow's expertise was psychology, his model represents progression in the mental/emotional realm. (These needs are listed on the left side of the diagram.)

On the right side of this diagram are the seven major energy centers. Just as acupuncture works to release blockages in unseen energy flow through channels called meridians, so the energy centers represent energy flow that cannot be easily seen or measured. They are depicted as vortices within specific regions of the body, pulling in energy from the larger field surrounding us.

Imagine that we could "plug into" external energy the way an appliance plugs into an electrical outlet. In this analogy, energy flows to us from an outside source, fills us, and allows us to use as much as

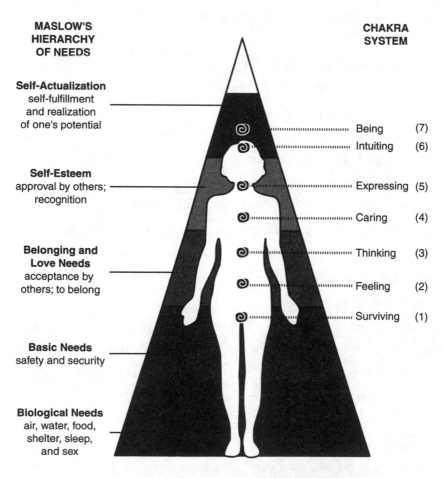

MASLOW'S HIERARCHY OF NEEDS

Self-Actualization
self-fulfillment and realization of one's potential

Self-Esteem
approval by others; recognition

Belonging and Love Needs
acceptance by others; to belong

Basic Needs
safety and security

Biological Needs
air, water, food, shelter, sleep, and sex

CHAKRA SYSTEM

Being (7)
Intuiting (6)
Expressing (5)
Caring (4)
Thinking (3)
Feeling (2)
Surviving (1)

Actualizing Our Healing Potential
© Karilee Halo Shames, R.N., Ph.D., H.N.C.

we need. As long as we're plugged into the source of energy, we have an infinite supply.

As long as our energy centers are open and flowing, we have input, throughput, and output in a continuous flow. However, when one or more energy centers becomes partially blocked, there is a diminished flow resulting in lack of energy and decreased capacity to be effective, leading eventually to "dis-ease."

Our challenge, as clients and healers, is to actualize our greatest potential. We can do this by allowing energy to flow freely through us, maximizing our physical, emotional, mental, and spiritual aspects of well-being.

The Major Energy Centers

The seven major energy centers or chakras correlate closely with Maslow's hierarchy of needs.

- The first energy center is at the base of the spine. It relates to survival and vitality.
- The second, just below the navel, relates to sexuality, creativity, and emotions.
- The third, in the solar plexus region above the navel, addresses fear and power issues, along with clear decision making.
- The heart center is known as "the great transformer," pulling energy up from the lower three centers (physical) into the higher realms (spiritual).
- The fifth energy center relates to communication and self-expression. It is situated in the thyroid area of the neck.
- The sixth is known in yogic philosophy as the "third eye." It facilitates clear-seeing or clairvoyance and is located in the region of the mid-forehead.

• The seventh center, at the very top of the skull, is known as the crown. This is where we interface with the Universal Energy Field, our Higher Power, or God, depending upon one's frame of reference.

Practical Examples of Energy Healing

When an energy center is blocked, the effect is similar to a buildup of debris in a creek: little by little, more debris accumulates, caught by the existing blockage until eventually there may be no water flowing at all. Depending upon which energy center is diminished, a variety of physical and emotional symptoms may result. Thus, it helps to keep your energy channels fully open.

Visual Meditation Number One—"Tap the Source of Healing Energy"
One of the most powerful strategies ever developed for boosting vitality involves the conscious directing of universal force into the energy centers. If you combine the enormous energy of the planet that supports you physically with the limitless power of universal mind, the results can be astounding. Below is an imagery meditation that we frequently use ourselves and highly recommend to our patients.

Sit comfortably in a chair. Take several moments to breathe deeply and become more relaxed. Feel your feet firmly planted on the floor, and let them grow warm as they connect you with the earth. With your eyes closed, imagine earth energy rising up through your feet, ankles, knees, thighs, and into your tailbone, the level of the first energy center. This is the center of survival and basic needs. See this center begin to glow with a warm red color as you pull up earth energy into it.

Observe as the area becomes brighter and brighter. Focus your attention on it until gradually it is filled with red light and glows in all directions. You will feel more and more comfortable as you continue to fill this center with light and realize that your physical safety and security are more assured with each breath. You are taken care of, protected, and loved.

Now, watch the light as it travels a short distance up to the level of your second energy center. This is the area related to sexuality, reproduction, and emotions. Here we also have connections based on sympathy and empathy.

See this center and your entire pelvic region gradually take on an orange glow, and continue to focus on it until it sparkles and radiates out in all directions. Only when it is fully saturated with warm glowing energy drawn up from the earth do you then move further upward.

You now see your third energy center, often considered to be near the solar plexus region, just above the navel. This is your center of fear and power, as well as of decision making. See this area bathed in a brilliant yellow energy drawn from the very center of the earth. When it is glowing brightly, and intensely radiating, move up to the heart, the fourth center.

The heart or the fourth energy center is our center of pure love. It is also "the great transformer," for here the earth energy from below can meet the vast heavenly energy from above. Breathe in a brilliant green, affirming your powerful ability to forgive and love. The fourth center is now glowing brightly, shining outward in all directions, radiating so gloriously that it appears to be spinning.

Enjoying this warmth, move up now to the neck and throat area. The fifth energy center controls communication and expression. As you focus on this area, envision a beautiful blue color, as if the sky were entering you, glowing and warming your vocal cords and thyroid area. See yourself communicating more openly, more effectively, and with greater enjoyment. Now imagine this blue area radiating in all directions.

Once your throat area is filled with a blue glow, move to the sixth center, between and slightly above your eyebrows. This area, known as the "third eye," allows for clairvoyance or clear vision. Activating this center, filling it with a beautiful indigo light, helps one to see clearly, with "all eyes" open. Fill this area with vibrant color until it is radiant. Affirm now your ability to see things more clearly.

Then move your focus even higher, to the crown of your head. This, the highest energy center, is the doorway to heaven, allowing connection to our Higher Power or God, our inner guidance and the wisdom of the Ages. This is the area of all-knowing, where universal light may enter and gather within us.

Envision this area as if there were a funnel above your head, drawing in pure radiant knowledge and energy from all of Creation. All the colors merge into a lustrous white glow that fills your entire being and emanates to those around you. You are vibrant, filled with life force. You are healthy and whole.

Let earth and sky meet within you. Be bathed in the flow of universal love and see your entire being filled with radiant white light. Let each organ and cell be open to this deepest sense of connection.

You are now tapping the true source of healing energy. This is the basic drive in living matter to balance and improve itself. See all the body systems coming into greater harmony with each other. Feel the vigor of what is now beyond energy and is rather a gathering of energies known as synergy. Especially experience an immune system that is more relaxed and discriminating. See it at peace with the rest of the body, which is now more fully alive than ever before.

From this place of power, feet firmly planted on the ground, begin to move back into waking awareness, using the energy gathered here to further your goals and visions.

Practice this meditation several times each week, if you like, until eventually it becomes a part of your waking affirmation.

Visual Meditation Number Two—"Laying On of Hands"
Pyramids in Egypt contain drawings from five thousand years ago, showing a person positioning his or her hands near another person's body, with wavy lines apparently depicting energy transmission. Laying on of hands is an ancient form of healing that has enjoyed wide use and that continues to be used even today across the world.

In this next visual meditation you will use your hands as well as your imagination to focus on healing of your thyroid area.

Sit comfortably in a chair. Take a few moments to breathe more deeply and allow yourself to become more relaxed. With your eyes closed, imagine the bottom of each foot drawing earth energy and wisdom up into your lower centers. Next imagine energy from high above descending into the body's upper centers. Envision in your mind's eye all of the energy centers lined up and working smoothly.

Focus now on the throat region at the base of the neck. Using both hands, gently stroke upward from your lowest center, bringing healing energy from the earth and the lower centers up to the throat area.

You can begin by gently stroking your body several times in an upward fashion. Then allow your hands to move an inch or two away from your body, while continuing to gently and slowly stroke upward.

After several upward strokes, reverse the process, now stroking downward from the top of the head. After several downward strokes, allow the hands to come to rest over the lower neck, comfortably cupping the thyroid area. Feel healing energy come through the hands and into the thyroid gland, revitalizing and nourishing it.

Imagine the thyroid now filled with healing energy, doing its job optimally. The thyroid hormones are in their proper ratios, and your chemical balance is now restored. Notice how good it feels to achieve this kind of harmony and vitality.

At this point, begin listening to your thyroid. Let it speak to you in pictures, symbols, feelings, or words. Consider any information you receive to be of high quality and primary importance.

Now establish a two-way communication between your highest consciousness and this vital organ. Ask what you can be doing to feel better more of the time, and consider examining various aspects of your life to determine which are serving you well, and which are not. Tell your thyroid that you will be taking better care of it from now on. Let it know that you will be paying closer attention to it on a regular basis, in the future.

Now, with several more deep cleansing breaths, begin to move back into waking awareness, having given caring healing attention to a most important body area.

These are but two examples of many powerful ways to maximize your health and well-being, using energy field concepts. We highly recommend them to you, whether you have an already diagnosed thyroid problem, or want to prevent its occurrence.

Integration—Bringing It All Together

Armed with the understanding we've outlined above, our clients often begin to relate to their symptoms in a bold new manner. Symptoms can be wakeup calls to return to the basics, to listen to the body. When one asks oneself, "What is my body trying to tell me?," answers may come in a variety of ways.

Some people keep journals, which allow them to write freely and brainstorm the personal meaning of their dis-ease. Others record meaningful dreams that they are then able to use in making greater sense of their lives. Many engage in some form of self-hypnosis or meditation, allowing them to access images and sensations that bridge the inner and outer worlds.

The Fully Actualized Health Care Consumer
The healing arts have made tremendous progress in recent years, sometimes by bridging Eastern religious mysticism and modern Western science. There is now a growing body of research demonstrating the health effects of these holistic interventions. In fact, we

live in a fascinating time of upheaval, chaos, and change. New ideas are being presented that challenge the medical establishment. This entrenched institution at first tries to resist the new techniques, but as they gradually prove useful, the establishment embraces them as its own.

Ideas that previously caused eyebrows to be raised are now being incorporated into standard practice. Those courageous enough to speak up for less costly and less invasive therapies are now no longer small voices in the dark but part of a major movement.

Nonetheless, it is up to health consumers to do more of their own homework. Consider all the data you can find about options and practitioners. Ask intelligent questions. Demand respect in a health care system that is undergoing enormous transformation.

Review both conventional and alternative research cautiously, for while it may be presented as gospel, more often than not there is a bias that interferes with objectivity. Find out who is funding or performing the research. Sometimes the company that stands the most to gain from a particular research result is the one funding, designing, and conducting experiments. While the experiments are presented as solid science, they certainly are not unbiased. This caveat can apply to claims made for health food items as well as for pharmaceuticals.

Remember that the voice of consumers is crucial if we are to co-create a healthy system. Important changes have occurred in hospitals because the consumers of health care have asked for them. For instance, natural birthing practices, availability of healers in operating rooms, more nutritious food choices, and parents being able to stay overnight with children are just some of the changes directly resulting from consumer input.

Thyroid as a Paradigm for Other Healing

Keep in mind the connection between thyroid healing and self-expression. Use your voice, speak your truth, and allow your inner wisdom to bring more peace and clarity to the world.

Marginal thyroid management is just one example of the suboptimal attention given by our critical-care medical system to people who suffer with chronic conditions. We hope this book can help all health consumers find a stronger voice for better treatment.

All of our voices are needed to inspire a transformation and revitalization in health care. As you strive to heal yourself, you are participating in a larger vision: the healing of the planet. Such participation is the essence of high level wellness and true vitality.

May your journey toward self-actualization be blessed with success, and may your example help others to heal along the way. May you touch many lives with your inspiration, and may the infinite life force be with you always.

How to Begin Your Program Quickly

While we generally recommend that thyroid changes occur in the gradual and stepwise fashion outlined so far, we realize some low thyroid sufferers want to "jump right in" and begin as quickly as possible. If this is more your style, we suggest starting as follows:

- *DAY ONE* See if you are a candidate for our ten-step thyroid improvement program. Take the questionnaire on page 19 (one out of every twelve people has some form of mild thyroid problem, and one out of every six older women). Find out if your fatigue, mood, weight, or other annoying symptoms make you part of this growing epidemic. If so, prepare to have your life changed for the better—low thyroid is easily treated.

If you are already taking either natural or prescription products, your score on the questionnaire may indicate areas of additional benefit possible with additional steps in our program. Also on this first day, you might go to the drugstore and purchase a mercury basal thermometer. Starting tomorrow, you can begin collecting five days' worth of morning readings. A low basal temperature is another piece of diagnostic evidence, indicating the need for further attention to your thyroid function. (See instructions for temperature test on page 268.)

- *DAY TWO* Generate a list of your definite medical and low-energy conditions, as well as any general tendencies to ill health. Be prepared for a shock. If you have low thyroid and start treating it optimally, your blood pressure, blood sugar, high cholesterol, irritable bowel, joint pain, skin problems—any or all of them—may dramatically improve. (Be sure to record your basal temperature from this morning.) Also on this second day order for yourself some of the best and strongest multivitamins with minerals (see Resources). In addition, purchase a bottle of mixed amino acids and a bottle of essential fatty acids. Take the label-recommended dose of each, and your thyroid may start feeling better right away. But don't stop here. There is much more to do.

- *DAY THREE* Talk to the relatives. Do people in your family have any gray hair before age thirty? dyslexia or attention deficit? carpal tunnel syndrome? mitral valve prolapse? white areas on the skin called vitiligo? Patchy hair loss called alopecia? anemia (a decrease in red blood cells), especially the pernicious or B_{12} type? left-handedness? manic depression? autoimmune problems

such as diabetes or rheumatoid arthritis? Especially question the
family about past or present low thyroid (some folks don't even
bother mentioning it as a medical problem because it is so common). Write down what they say. It is all part of your ticket to a
life-changing diagnosis. Fill out the questionnaire at the end of
Step 3 and arrange to show your point total to your health care
provider. Resolve today to be more proactive and empowered
when dealing with the medical establishment. Remember that
you are the captain of your own ship, and you need to forge
ahead unwaveringly on what you feel is the best course for you.

- ***DAY FOUR*** Check your home medical records or make a
  phone call to see if you've had any thyroid blood tests in the
  last few years. (Thyroid blood tests are generally listed on print-
  outs as T-4 or T-3U or FTI or FT4.) If your testing did not
  include a TSH level, ask to have that test ordered for you now.
  If you had a TSH test and were told it was normal, check now
  for the exact number. If the actual result was 2.5 or above, you
  may not be so normal after all. At this point ask to have some
  additional thyroid blood tests ordered (see Step 4). Also on this
  fourth day, make a commitment to start right now decreasing
  your exposure to artificial chemicals in your food, air, and water.
  These may be mild immune triggers for you, silently affecting
  your thyroid function. In addition, resolve today to henceforth
  avoid anything that has ever before caused you an allergic
  response, even a mild one. Continue recording your early
  morning temperature, and keep taking your new supplements.

- ***DAY FIVE*** If you are not already taking thyroid medication,
  become acquainted with the wide range of options (several over-

the-counter types, and several prescription varieties). Find out which work best for your friends or family and which mesh well with your own beliefs and lifestyle. If you are already taking thyroid medicine, ask yourself if it is as effective as you would like, or if there might be some improvement. (Sometimes a change of dose or a mixture of items will work better than what you are currently taking). Compile an average of basal temperatures over the last four days. If you average below 97.8 or if you have scored high on the questionnaires, here is something you can start doing immediately. Regardless of any thyroid medications or supplements you might be taking currently, you may right now purchase one of several thyroid glandular—supports (see Resources). Start by taking one pill a day for the next few weeks and begin feeling better. Continue to expand and refine your program with additional suggestions from the ten steps and additional ideas from your health providers.

- *AFTER THE FIFTH DAY* Now that you have gotten a jump start on your thyroid program, you can easily keep this momentum going. Start talking to friends about your thyroid interests. Compare notes with people at work and on the Internet. Elicit their support, feedback, and suggestions, because group effort is more effective than isolation in tackling this particular issue. Take one minute each evening to sit comfortably with your eyes closed, and listen to what your thyroid may want to tell you. All of this will help create a new and more positive attitude.

- *INTO THE FUTURE* The 5-Day Jump Start is just one quick way to begin using your stepwise thyroid program. You need not follow every single suggestion we have mentioned.

Nor must you approach the steps in the exact order presented. Try things out, see what works for you. Continue to build your own individualized version of thyroid recovery.

You might find it surprisingly satisfying to work on more than one level at once (see Step 10). This could take the form of addressing physical needs and psychological needs together, or psychological and spiritual needs simultaneously. Consider the musician who plays a guitar. If each string is well tuned, each will make a satisfactory sound. When all three are played together, a harmonious chord will result, creating a richer, fuller, and more vibrant sound. It is here that the exquisite subtlety of music can truly emerge.

Perhaps you have known occasions when your life has struck such a resonant chord. It occurs when the physical, mental, and spiritual realms are synchronized and are all working together.

Always keep in mind that thyroid health is a journey, and not a destination. Regardless of how fast you get started, be at ease with however long the process of regaining your health is taking. Cures of a lasting nature, like any enduring change, take place in their own time and at their own speed. Many people, for instance, are in such a hurry to lose weight quickly that they spend years losing and regaining, losing and regaining. To get beyond this frustrating rhythm, make each change easy enough that you could live with it forever. Be comforted in knowing that you have begun to take the proper steps and are on a meaningful path.

Finally, be gentle with yourself. In this difficult world, you have done quite well to be where you are today. Allow for more enjoyment of your present state of wholeness. From this wellspring of increased acceptance and harmonious living flows more of the healing you seek. We wish you great success on your journey.

Show This to Your Doctor

Dear Doctor:

Your patient has read my book on autoimmune hypothyroidism and wants to share it with you. I am a Harvard, University of Pennsylvania, and NIH-trained primary care physician. After thirty years of largely endocrine practice, including management of several of my own family members with this condition, I now better understand the extensive morbidity that even mild thyroiditis can cause. This book combines some favorite clinical pearls with a preventive medicine literature search. (See list of thyroid articles in Further Reading.) Each chapter is a separate step to motivate the health care consumer. Here is a medical version of the steps, along with an abbreviated literature rationale:

Step 1. **New studies suggest a surprisingly high incidence of borderline hypothyroidism.**

- "The symptoms associated with mild thyroid failure may not be apparent to the clinician. The incidence of mild hypothyroidism in the U.S. is about 10% . . . 20% in older women." Ridgeway, E. C., *Hypothyroidism: The Hidden Challenge*, Clinical Management Conference Statement (Denver: University of Colorado School of Medicine, 1996): 4.

- "In reality, about 25% of individuals do seem to have . . . the unfortunate capacity to make antibodies to fragments of some of their own body cells." Wood, Lawrence C., *Your Thyroid* (New York: Ballantine Books, 1995): 26.

Step 2. **Coexistent subclinical hypothyroidism often exacerbates other disease symptomatology.**

- "Thyroiditis is a commonly overlooked problem in perhaps 10% of chronically ill patients. Appropriate treatment with thyroid medication can be immensely helpful for many of them. I strongly recommend always getting thyroid antibodies as part of the initial workup." Wilkinson, R., M.D., "Thyroid Dysfunction and Treatment," CME monograph (Tucson, University of Arizona School of Medicine, 1997).

- "Autoimmune thyroid patients show high prevalence of autoantibody to nonthyroid antigens and organs." Morita, S. et al., "Prevalence of Non-Thyroid Specific Auto-antibodies in Autoimmune Thyroid Disease," *J Clin Endocrinol Metab* 80, no. 4 (1995):1203–1206.

Step 3. **Accurate diagnosis of mild hypothyroidism requires a detailed history and a high index of suspicion.**

- "The decision to initiate therapy should be based on both

clinical and laboratory findings, and not solely on the results of a single laboratory test." Sachs, B., *Thyroid*, vol. 3, no. 4 (1993): 353–354.

- "The bulk of relevant information can be obtained from a carefully gathered history and meticulously executed physical—a battery of tests must not replace a mind willing to question." Lown, Bernard, *The Lost Art of Healing* (New York: Houghton Mifflin, 1996).

Step 4. Standard thyroid tests have a disturbingly high rate of false negatives.

- ". . . [a long list of thyroid lab tests] . . . did not, except in patients with gross abnormalities, distinguish euthyroid patients from those who were receiving inadequate or excessive replacement. These measurements are therefore of little, if any, value in monitoring patients receiving thyroxine replacement." Fraser, W., et al., "Are Biochemical Tests of Thyroid Function of Any Value in Monitoring Patients Receiving Thyroxine Replacement?" *Br Med J* (Clin Res Ed) (September 27, 1997): 293 (6550): 808–810.

- "Even if the highly-sensitive TSH is in the lower segment of the normal range, a person may still be suffering from low-grade hypothyroidism." Arem, Ridha, M.D., Associate Professor of Endocrinology at Baylor University, *The Thyroid Solution* (New York: Ballantine Books, 1999).

Step 5. No single method of thyroid replacement is optimal for all patients.

- "Partial substitution of triiodothyronine for thyroxine may improve mood and neuropsychological function." Bunevicius, R. et al., "Effects of Thyroxine As Compared with Thyroxine

Plus Triiodothyronine in Patients with Hypothyroidism,"
New England Journal of Medicine 340, no.6 (February 11,
1999):424–491.

- "Treatment of Hashimoto's Thyroiditis requires lifelong
administration of thyroid hormone to correct or prevent
hypothyroidism. The common replacement is 125–175 mcg.
of thyroxine (with or without T3). Many of my patients do
better with Armour." Wilkinson, R., M.D., "Thyroid Dysfunction and Treatment," CME monograph (Tucson, University of Arizona School of Medicine, 1997).

**Step 6. Mild thyroid failure can result in, or masquerade as,
reproductive hormone imbalance.**

- "Thyroid dysfunction frequently occurs after delivery through
an immune rebound mechanism. Laboratory tests in the postpartum period are essential to diagnose post-partum onset of
autoimmune disease . . ." Hidaka, Y., "Post-Partum Depression or Post-Partum Thyroiditis?" Department of Laboratory
Medicine, Osaka University Medical School. *Rinsho Byori* 43,
no.11 (November 1995):1107-1109.

- "Severe menopause is just one of the early symptomatic end-
points of borderline low thyroid." Feit, H., "Thyroid Function in the Elderly," *Clin Ger Med* 4 (1988): 151–161.

**Step 7. Adverse hormonal sequelae of autoimmunity can
include hypofunction of adrenal as well as thyroid tissues.**

- "We have determined a significant coexistence of autoimmune thyroid disorders in patients with Addison's Disease.
The autoimmune mechanism was the most probable cause of
adrenocortical insufficiency in most patients." Kasperlik-
Zaluska, A., "High Prevalence of Thyroid Autoimmunity in

Idiopathic Addison's Disease," *Autoimmunity* 18, no.3 (1994): 213–216.

- "Physiologic doses of hydrocortisone acetate may increase T3 receptor function and in such small amounts may actually improve the peripheral conversion of T4 into T3." Jeffries, W., *Safe Uses of Cortisone* (Springfield, IL: Charles Thomas Publisher, 1991):155–157.

Step 8. Malnutrition can retard the restoration of optimal thyroid function.

- "Thyroid patients should be on multivitamins and multiminerals. They may need extra iron, and folic acid orally, along with B_{12} by injection." Wilkinson, R., M.D., "Thyroid Dysfunction and Treatment," CME monograph (Tucson: University of Arizona School of Medicine, 1997).
- "Proper nutrition is essential for optimal endocrine system balance." Frame, P., "A Critical Review of Adult Health Maintenance. Part 4. Prevention of Metabolic, Behavioral, and Miscellaneous Conditions." *J Pharm Prac* 23 (1986):29–39.

Step 9. Hormone replacement that yields a low-normal TSH is only one way to decrease the autoimmune pressure on the pituitary-thyroid axis.

- "The prevalence of coexisting celiac and thyroid disease . . . was significantly more than expected. This association is clinically important . . . the coexistence of the two conditions led to diagnostic difficulties and delay of treatment." Counsell, C. et al., "Coexistence of Celiac and Thyroid Disease." *Gut 35*, no.6 (1994): 844–846.
- "Remissions in autoimmune thyroid disease may occur via factors that modulate thyroid cell activity, thereby reducing

thyrocyte-immunocyte signaling." Volpe, R., "Autoimmunity
Causing Thyroid Dysfunction," *Endocrinol Metab Clin North
Am* 20, no.3 (September 1991): 565–587.

**Step 10. Chances of optimal recovery are improved with
healthier lifestyle behaviors.**

- "An activated patient is both desirable and possible in light of
new advances in habit modification." Bartalena, L., "Cigarette
Smoking and the Thyroid," *Eur J Endocrinol* 133, no.5
(November 1995): 507–512.

- "Several different non-genetic risk factors are of importance in
[autoimmune hormone disease] . . . early exposure to cow's
milk protein and a high frequency of intake of nitrosamine-
rich food . . . exposure to many infectious diseases, a cold
environment, and stressful life events, may promote an
already ongoing autoimmune destructive process . . ."
Dahlquist, G., "Non-Genetic Risk Factors in Autoimmune
Endocrine Disease," *Diabete Metab*. 20, no. 3 (May–June
1999):251–257.

In closing, I would like to thank you for taking the time from
your busy schedule to review this line of reasoning. I wish for you and
your patient a mutually beneficial experience.

Kindest regards to you both,
Richard L. Shames, M.D.

Useful Terms

Amiodarone: A heart drug that contains iodine and has been found to trigger the onset of both high and low thyroid.

Armour Thyroid: Brand name for natural (nonsynthetic) thyroid hormone, made with desiccated animal thyroid gland, usually from pigs.

Attention Deficit Disorder: Learning disability that involves difficulty concentrating on a task at hand. This condition has been associated with low thyroid disorders.

Autoantibody: A protein chemical made by immune system B-cells, wrongly programmed to attack one's own tissues.

Autoimmunity: A situation in which a person's immune system makes autoantibodies in any significant degree.

Basal Body Temperature: A person's temperature taken first thing in the morning, before arising from bed, usually measured with a basal thermometer, placed in the center of the bare armpit; a useful indicator of one's basal metabolic rate, which is generally low in hypothyroid conditions.

Bone Density Test: A laboratory evaluation using mild external radiation to determine the amount of calcium in bone. Lower levels are related to increased risk of fracture.

Borderline Low Thyroid: Decreased output of thyroid hormone from the thyroid gland; also called mild thyroid failure; frequently too mild to result in severe symptoms or obviously abnormal lab tests, but often severe enough to be life-limiting in some way; *see* Subclinical Hypothyroidism.

Chronic Lymphocytic Thyroiditis: Also known as Hashimoto's Disease, this is a disorder characterized by autoimmune attack on the thyroid gland, the most common cause of low thyroid function.

Cytomel: Brand name for prescription medicine made with synthetic triiodothyronine (T-3, the rapid-acting thyroid hormone);

used to treat low thyroid conditions by itself or more recently, in combination with thyroxine (T-4, the slow-acting thyroid hormone).

Desiccated Thyroid: The generic name for tablets of animal thyroid gland used to treat low thyroid conditions; its active ingredients include both T-3 and T-4 (brand names include Armour, Westroid, Naturthroid, and Proloid).

Endocrine Disruptors: Unwanted chemicals in the environment that block, alter, or mimic the function of normal endocrine hormones or disrupt endocrine glands.

Euthroid: Brand name of a prescription medicine, similar to Thyrolar; no longer commonly available.

Euthyroid: The state of normal thyroid function, per blood test determination.

Fine Needle Aspiration: A common way of performing a biopsy on the thyroid gland, using a thin needle.

Free T-4: Thyroxine (slow-acting thyroid hormone) that is not bound to transport proteins in the bloodstream.

Free T-3: Thyronine (rapid-acting thyroid hormone) that is not bound to transport proteins in the bloodstream.

Goiter: An enlargement, or swelling, of the thyroid gland.

Goitrogen: A chemical, or food, that causes a goiter in the thyroid gland.

Hashimoto's Disease: Autoimmune inflammation of the thyroid gland, named for the Japanese doctor who first described it. It is the most common cause of simple low thyroid function.

Hormone Disruptor: A chemical in the air, food, or water that confuses or disrupts normal hormone function.

Hormones: Chemicals made in the body (or taken as medicines) that are carried in the bloodstream to various organs, thereby affecting body functions.

Hypothyroidism: Insufficient production of thyroid hormone due to abnormal thyroid gland function, absence of all or some of the thyroid gland, or lack of sufficient thyroid hormone medication.

Iodine: A chemical element found in seafood and sea salt, and added to most table salt; essential nutrient necessary for the body's capacity to make thyroid hormone. In too high a dose, it inhibits the body's ability to make thyroid hormone.

Levothroid: Brand name for prescription medicine made with synthetic thyroxine (T-4, the slow-acting thyroid hormone). It is of high quality and color coded according to dosage.

Levothyroxine: Generic term referring to T-4, the slow-acting thyroid hormone (also called l-thyroxine).

Levoxyl: Brand name for prescription medicine made with synthetic thyroxine (T-4, the slow-acting thyroid hormone); it is of high quality and is available in the form of easily breakable diamond-shaped tablets useful for fine-tuning the dose.

L-Thyroxine: A shortened way to write levothyroxine.

Microsomal Antibody Test: A blood test used to ascertain the presence of autoimmunity to the thyroid gland (*see* Peroxidase Antibody Test).

Natural Thyroid: Nonsynthetic, animal-derived thyroid hormone (*see* Desiccated Thyroid).

Osteoporosis: A frequently mild condition of bone loss, especially from the hip and spine, causing (in severe stages) a greater likelihood of fracture.

Peroxidase Antibody Test: The same as, but more sensitive than, the microsomal antibody test.

Postpartum Thyroiditis: Autoimmune inflammation of the thyroid gland occurring after pregnancy; frequently a cause of postpartum depression.

Receptor: A complex chemical site on or inside cells; it is to the receptor that messenger molecules, such as hormones, will bind and create some specific action in the target cell.

Reverse T-3: A form of triiodothyronine (T-3, the rapid-acting thyroid hormone) that is manufactured during times of body stress and during certain illnesses. Reverse T-3 is an inactive thyroid hormone.

Selenium: A mineral important in the production and function of thyroid hormone; its adequate supplementation is encouraged for thyroid sufferers.

Subclinical Hypothyroidism: Decreased output of thyroid hormone from the thyroid gland, too mild to result in obvious symptoms or grossly abnormal blood tests, but possibly severe enough to be life-limiting in some way (*see* Borderline Low Thyroid).

Suppressor T-Cell: A member of the lymphocyte family of white blood cells, matured in the thymus gland—hence the letter T—this cell helps balance the immune system by decreasing previously started immune activity.

Synthroid: Brand name for prescription medicine made with synthetic thyroxine (T-4, the slow-acting thryoid hormone); the most common of the synthetic thyroids; it has been the second most frequently prescribed medication in the United States.

T-Cell: A white blood cell in the lymphocyte family involved in cellular immunity.

Thyroglobulin Antibody Test: A blood test used to determine the presence of autoimmunity against the thyroid system.

Thyroiditis: General term for thyroid inflammation, usually used as the short name for Hashimoto's autoimmune thyroiditis; the term is also used in several other specific kinds of thyroid inflammation syndromes.

Thyrolar: Brand name for prescription medication made with a fixed-ratio mixture of synthetic T-3 and T-4 (respectively the rapid-acting and the slow-acting thyroid hormones).

T-3 (Triiodothyronine): Rapid-acting thyroid hormone, each molecule containing three atoms of iodine; it performs its job by attaching to the binding site inside body cells, thereby affecting DNA function in the cell nucleus.

T-4 (Thyroxine): Slow-acting thyroid hormone, each molecule containing four atoms of iodine; needs to be converted to T-3 in the body before attaching to the binding site inside body cells and affecting DNA function in the cell nucleus.

Thyrotropin: Another name for thyroid stimulating hormone (*see* TSH).

TRH (Thyrotropin Releasing Hormone): A brain messenger molecule secreted by the hypothalamus to regulate the amount of TSH released by the pituitary.

TRH Test: An extremely sensitive thyroid function test that can detect borderline or mild hypothyroidism when other tests, including a sensitive TSH test, show normal.

TSH (Thyroid Stimulating Hormone): A pituitary gland hormone secreted to regulate function of the thyroid gland.

Articles on the Fluoride-Thyroid Connection

For more information, contact the Fluoride Action Network (www.fluoride alert.org). as well as Andreas Schuld (www.bruha.com/fluoride).

Our Top Three Highly Recommended Articles

1. Colquhoun, J. "Why I Changed My Mind About Water Fluoridation," from the prestigious, peer-reviewed journal of the University of Chicago. *Perspectives in Biology and Medicine* 41, no. 1: (Autumn 1997). Reprinted by Safe Water Information Service, 1998.

   Dr. Colquhoun was Principal Dental Officer in Auckland, New Zealand, and a former advocate of fluoridation. He studied all local dental decay rates, then embarked on a world tour to prove the efficacy of fluoridation but learned many disturbing facts and reversed his position.

2. Hirzy, J. W. "Why EPA Headquarters Union of Scientists Opposes Fluoridation," May 1, 1999. Open Letter from National Treasury Employees Union, Chapter 280, Washington D.C.

    Explains why the Environmental Protection Agency, representing 1,500 scientists, lawyers, and engineers, took a stand in opposing fluoridation of drinking water supplies. Includes concerns about dental fluorosis (mottling of teeth), impaired pineal function, gene mutations, cancer, reproduction effects, neurotoxicity, and bone pathology. Cites major references, some included on the list below. Dr. Hirzy can be reached at hirzy.john@epa.gov.

3. Natick Fluoridation Study Committee. "Should Natick Fluoridate?" A Summary of the Report to the Town and the Board of Selectmen (1997).

    This document describes the findings of the selectmen of a Massachusetts town, who studied carefully and reviewed the literature, eventually concluding that the potential harm from fluoridation was greater than the potential advantages.

Our Top Recommended Book

Yiamouyiannis, J. *Fluoride: The Aging Factor*. Delaware, OH: Health Action Press, 1993.

    Excellent book detailing biochemistry and politics of fluoride.

Other Helpful Articles

Balabolkin, M. I. et al. "The interrelationship of the thyroid and immune statuses of workers with long-term fluorine exposure." *Ter Arkh* 67(1): 41–2 (1995).

Day, T. K. and P. R. Powell-Jackson. "Fluoride, water hardness, and endemic goitre." *Lancet* 1:1135–1138 (1972).

Fejerskov, O., F. Manji, V. Baelum. "The nature and mechanisms of dental fluorosis in man." *J Dent Res* 69 spec no: 692–700; discussion 721 (1990) Department of Oral Anatomy, Dental Pathology, and Operative Dentistry, Royal Dental College, Aarhus, Denmark.

Galetti, P. M. and G. Joyet. "Effect of fluorine on thyroidal iodine metabolism in hyperthyroidism." *J Clin Endocrinol* 18:1102–10 (1958).

Grimbergen, G. W. "A double blind test for determination of intolerance to fluoridated water (preliminary report)," *Fluoride* 7:146–52 (1974).

Hillman, D., D. L. Bolenbaugh, E. M. Convey. "Hypothyroidism and anemia related to fluoride in dairy cattle." *J Dairy Sci* 62(3): 416–23 (1979).

Huda, S. N. et al. "Biochemical hypothyroidism secondary to iodine deficiency is associated with poor school achievement and cognition in Bangladeshi children." *Journal of Nutrition* 129(5): 980–87 (1999).

Judd, G. "Good teeth birth to death," Research Publications, Glendale, AZ (1997), EPA Research #2 (1994).

Kunzel, V. W. "Cross-sectional comparison of the median eruption time for permanent teeth in children from fluoride poor and optimally fluoridated areas." *Stomatol DDR* 5:310–21 (1976).

Li, X. S., J. L. Zhi, and R. O. Gao. "Effect of fluoride exposure on intelligence in children." *Fluoride* 28 (1995).

Luke, J. A. "Effect of fluoride on the physiology of the pineal gland." *Caries Research* 28:204 (1994).

Roholm, K. "fluorine intoxication—a clinical hygiene study, with a review of the literature and some experimental investigations." H. K. Lewis & Co., London (1937).

Schlesinger, E. R. et al. "Newburgh-Kingston caries-fluorine study XIII. Pediatric findings after 10 years." *JADA* 52: 296–306 (1956).

Sherrell, D. "Documentation of rising intake of fluorides"—26 official documents compiled by Darlene Sherrell, Dental Fluorosis Prevention Program. http://www.riv.net/-fluoride/riseinta.htm.

Spira, L. "The drama of fluorine—arch enemy of mankind." Milwaukee Press (1953) (compilation of published articles).

Spittle, B. "Allergy and hypersensitivity to fluoride." *Fluoride* 26: 267–273 (1993).

Wilson, R. H. and F. DeEds. "The synergistic action of thyroid on fluorine toxicity." *Endocrinology* 26:851 (1940).

Zhao, L. B. et al. "Effect of high fluoride water supply on children's intelligence." *Fluoride* 29:190–192 (1996).

Zhao, W. et al. "Long-term effects of various iodine and fluorine doses on the thyroid and fluorosis in mice." *Endocr Regul* 32(2):63–70 (1998).

Resources

Please feel free to contact the authors at their informational website: www.thyroidpower.com or call toll free 1-866-GoThyRx (1-866-468-4979).

Finding Practitioners

American Association of Clinical Endocrinologists
2589 Park Street
Jacksonville, FL 32204
(904) 384-9490
www.aace.com

American Holistic Medical Association
6728 Old McLean Village Drive
McLean, VA 22101
(703) 556-9728
www.holisticmedicine.org

American Holistic Nurses Association
P.O. Box 2130
Flagstaff, AZ 86003-2130
(800) 278-AHNA
www.ahna.org

Broda Barnes, M.D. Research Foundation
P.O. Box 98
Trumbull, CT 06611
(203) 261-2101
www.brodabarnes.org

Endocrine Society
4350 East West Highway, Suite 500
Bethesda, MD 20814
(301) 941-0200
www.endo-society.org

Thyroid Organizations

For organizations that offer highest quality nutritional products, the authors recommend that you contact their constantly updated clearinghouse for thyroid information and treatment called ThyRx. You can call toll free about products at (866) GO-THYRX or see www.thyroidpower.com for a listing of products and latest research.

American Autoimmune-Related Diseases Association
21200 Gratiot Avenue
Detroit, MI 48201
(800) 598-4668
www.aarda.org

American Foundation of Thyroid Patients
P.O. Box 820195
Houston, TX 77282
(888) 996-4460
www.thyroidfoundation.org

Endocrine Nurses Society
P.O. Box 229
West Linn, OR 97068
(503) 494-3714

Thyroid Foundation of America
Ruth Sleeper Hall, RSL 350
40 Parkman Street
Boston, MA 02114
(800) 832-8321
www.tfawed.org/pub/tfa

Thyroid Foundation of Canada
96 Mack Street
Kingston, Ontario, Canada K711N9
(613) 544-8364
www.thyroid-fed.org

Thyroid Society for Education and Research
7515 South Main Street, Suite 545
Houston, TX 77030
(713) 799-9909
www.the-thyroid-society.org

The MAGIC Foundation (Clinical Hypothyroid Division)
Thomas P. Foley, Jr., M.D.; Professor of Pediatrics, University of Pittsburgh and
    Children's Hospital of Pittsburgh, Pennsylvania: www.magicfoundation.org/
    clinhypop.html

Thyroid Websites

http://thyroid.miningco.com/blchklst.htm?pid=2750&cob=home
http://vesalius.cpmc.columbia.edu/texts/gcps/gcpsoo3o.html
http://home.ican.net/~thyroid/canada.html
http://thyroid.tqn.com/blchklst.html
www.med.stanford.edu/center/communications/Stanmed/Summer95/thyroid.html
www.digitalnation.com/mshomon/thyroid/
www.glandcentral.com
www.healthy.net/Library/Articles/Schacter/hypothyr.d.html
www.hsc.missouri.edu/medicine/thyroid/thy_dis.html
www.mayohealth.org/mayo/9409/htm/
www.thriveonline.com/health/Library/CAD/abstract11202.html
www.thyroid.miningco.com

Additional Related Organizations/Websites

Chronic Fatigue and Immune Dysfunction Syndrome Association
P.O. Box 220398
Charlotte, NC 28222
(800) 442-3437

Consortium for Environmental Education in Medicine
www.ceem/org/

Endocrine Disruptors
www.osf-facts.org

Endocrine Disruptors
www.wwfcanada.org/hormone-disruptors

Environmental Research Foundation
P.O. Box 5036
Annapolis, MD 21403
FAX: (415) 263-8944
Email: erf@rachel.org

Fact Sheets Chlorine, PVCÆs and Dioxins
www.Greenpeace.org

H.A.P.P.E.N. (Holistic Alliance of Professional Practitioners, Entrepreneurs, and
    Networkers)
P.O. Box 665
Black Mountain, NC 28711-0666
(888) 8HAPPEN
www.HAPPEN.org

Health Care Without Harm
www.sustain.org/hcwh

Indoor Air Quality
www.envirosense.org

Information Clearinghouse and Referral Center promoting Alternatives to Toxic
    chemicals
www.accessone.com/~watoxics

Mothers and Others for a Liveable Planet
www.mothers.org/mothers

National Foundation for Depressive Illness
P.O. Box 2257
New York, NY 10116
(800) 248-4344

Sustainable Alternatives to Pesticides
www.igc.org

Update and Dangers of Toxic and Endocrine-Disrupting Chemicals
www.monitor.net/Rachel/

(see Fluoride Facts for fluoride websites)

Special Laboratories for Hormone Testing

Aeron Lifecycles
(laboratory for saliva testing of hormones)
1933 Davis St., Suite 310
San Leandro, CA 94577
(800) 631-7900

Balco Clinical Laboratories
(mineral analysis of blood, hair, and urine)
1520 Gilbreth Road
Burlingame, CA 94010
(800) 777-7122

Broda Barnes, M.D. Research Foundation
(urine determination of thyroid status)
P.O. Box 98
Trumbull, CT 06611
(203) 261-2101

Corning-Nichols Diagnostic Laboratory
(special determinations for TSH antibodies)
33608 Ortega Highway
San Juan Capistrano, CA 92675
(800) NICHOLS

Diagnos-Techs, Inc.
(adrenal hormone testing)
P.O. Box 58948
Seattle, WA 98138
(206) 251-0596

Great Smokies Diagnostic Laboratory
(for parasite testing)
63 Zillicoa St., Asheville, NC 28801
(800) 522-4762

Immuno-Diagnostics Laboratory
(excellent lab for routine and special blood thyroid tests)
10930 Bigge Street
San Leandro, CA 94577
(800) 88-1113

Meridian Valley Clinical Laboratory
(all-around lab, especially for parasite testing)
515 West Harrison St., Suite 9
Kent, WA 98032
(800) 234-6825

Vitamin Diagnostics
(vitamin levels and urine determination of thyroid status)
Route 35 and Industrial Drive
Cliffwood Beach, NJ 07735
(732) 583-7773

Water Filtration Devices

There are a variety of good companies offering filtration devices for your home or office. A good carbon block filter can eliminate many chemicals, including chlorine. To eliminate fluoride, you need a reverse-osmosis or a distillation device. Our favorite filter company, which could also give you further information about other companies and products, is:

Multi-Pure Corporation
Las Vegas Technology Center
P.O. Box 34630
Las Vegas, NV 89133-4630
(800) 622-9206

Tests

Commonly Available Tests for Evaluating Low Thyroid Function (in order of simplicity and economy of cost)

- Basal temperature test
- Thyroid Stimulating Hormone (TSH)
- T-4 Panel
    Total T-4
    T-3 Uptake
    Free Thyroxine Index (FTI)
- T-3 Total
- Free T-3

- Free T-4
- Thyroglobulin level (Tg)
- Thyroxine-Binding Globulin (TBG)
- Antiperoxidase (Microsomal) Antibody Titer
- Antithyroglobulin Antibody Titer
- Thyroid urine test (available through Broda Barnes, M.D. Research Foundation and Vitamin Diagnostics—see Resources)
- TRH test
- Thyroid ultrasound
- Thyroid scan and radioactive iodine uptake (RAIU)
- Fine Needle Aspiration (FNA)

Our Suggested Panel of Thyroid Tests

(the minimum amount of testing we think is needed before you can be told, "It doesn't look like low thyroid is causing your symptoms")

- TSH
- Basal temperature test
- T-4 Panel (Total T-4, T-3 Uptake, Free Thyroxine Index)
- T-3 Total
- Antiperoxidase (microsomal) antibody

Adrenal Testing

Commonly Available Tests for Evaluating Low Adrenal Function (in order of simplicity and economy of cost)

- Cortisol levels (8 A.M. and 4 P.M.)
- Blood catecholamines
- DHEA and DHEA-S levels
- 24-hour urine (for catecholamines and fourteen ketosteroids)
- Adrenal Stress Index (ASI–urine)—four separate tests of urine Cortisol, taken at four different times during the day
- Adrenal Stress Index (ASI–saliva)—four separate tests of saliva Cortisol, taken at four different times during the day
- Cortrosyn stimulation test for adrenal reserve

Sex Hormone Testing

(commonly available tests for reproductive evaluation)

- Estrogen level (Total estrogens or estradiol level)
- Estrogen fractionation
    Estradiol level
    Estrone level
    Estriol level
    Total estrogens
- Progesterone level
- Total testosterone
- Free testosterone
- Follicle Stimulating Hormone (FSH)
- Luteinizing Hormone (LH)
- Prolactin

Medications Useful for Low Thyroid

Prescription

    T-4 (l-thyroxine)

      Synthroid

      Levoxyl

      Levothroid

      levothyroxine (generic)

    T-3 (thyronine or triiodothyronine)

      Cytomel

      Timed-release T-3

    T-3/T-4 combinations

      Thyrolar

Dessicated thyroid
   Armour
   Naturthroid
   Westroid
   generic

Over-the-Counter

Thyroid glandular (dessicated thyroid with active ingredients removed)
   Thyroid 130
   GF Thyroid
   Thyroplex
Thytrophin (nucleus material from thyroid cells)
Homeopathics
   Thyroid 6x (pellets)
   Thyroid R-6 (liquid)
   Thyroidium (various potencies)

Food Choices

Foods to Favor (Eat more of these)
- Fresh whole foods
- Simple organic foods (low in artificial or chemical content)
- Low-fat foods
- Good sources of protein
    Fish (deep sea or pond-raised)
    Meat (organic, range-fed; eat small amounts at a time, no more than one serving daily)
    Poultry (organic/free range, without hormones or chemicals)
- High complex carbohydrates
    Vegetables (squash, asparagus)

Grains (brown rice, oats)

Sprouts

Beans

Sweet potatoes

Foods to Avoid (Minimize or try to eliminate)
- "S.F.–C.A.T.S."
    salt

    fats

    caffeine

    alcohol

    tobacco

    sugar
- Fast foods
- Fried foods
- Trans-fats (hydrogenated vegetable oils)
- Goitrogens
    peanuts

    pine nuts

    cassava (tapioca)

    sorghum
- Aspartame (Equal/Nutrasweet)

Foods to Limit (one serving or less per day)
- Dairy products (eat low/nonfat, organic)
- Soy products
- Cruciferous vegetables (Brussels sprouts, cabbage, cauliflower, broccoli)

Our Suggested Daily Dosage for Hypothyroidism

See Resources for ease of purchase and quality assurance, author website, or call toll free 1-866-GoThyRx (1-866-468-4979)

Extra-Strength Multivitamin with Minerals

A	10,000–15,000 IU
C	250–500 mg
E	400–600 IU
B-complex	50–100 mg
Folic acid	400–800 mg
Copper	1–2 mg
Zinc	25–30 mg
Selenium	100–200 mg

Chromium	100–200 mg
Manganese	10–20 mg

Additional Antioxidants

Vitamin C	2,000 mg
Pygnogenol	100 mg
Lipoic acid	100 mg
Vitamin E	An additional 800–1,200 IU will help menopausal women reduce their hot flashes

Fatty Acids

Omega-6 (linoleic acid)	250 mg (especially evening primrose oil, a source of GLA)
Omega-3 (linolenic acid)	500 mg (especially flax oil, a source of EPA and DHA)

Amino Acids

Free-form aminos	1,000 mg
Extra tyrosine	500 mg
Extra Glutamine	500 mg

Herbal Support

Milk Thistle (silymarin, an antioxidant)	300 mg

Notes

Step 1: Consider Thyroid the Hidden Factor in Your Overall Health

1. E. C. Ridgeway, *Hypothyroidism: The Hidden Challenge*, monograph (University of Colorado School of Medicine, December 1996).
2. Lawrence C. Wood, *Your Thyroid* (New York: Ballantine Books, 1995): 26.
3. J. C. Galofre et al., "Incidence of Different Forms of Thyroid Dysfunction and Its Degrees in an Iodine Sufficient Area." *Thyroidology* 6, no.2 (1994): 49–54.

Step 2: Learn How Low Thyroid Makes Any Illness Worse

1. R. Hoffman, "Chronic Inflammation and Airway Disease," *Alternative & Complementary Therapies* (June/July 1995): 217.

2. K. Fukada et al., "The Chronic Fatigue Syndrome: A Comprehensive Approach to Its Definition and Study," *Annals of Internal Medicine* 121, no. 12 (1995): 626–631.

Step 3: Use Signs, Symptoms, and Family History to Support a Diagnosis

1. C. P. Barsano, "Other Forms of Primary Hypothyroidism," in *The Thyroid: A Fundamental Clinical Text*, 6th ed., L. E. Braverman and R. D. Utiger, eds., (Philadelphia, PA: J. B. Lippincott, 1991): 956–967.
2. M. T. Hays and K. R. K. Nielsen, "Human Thyroxin Absorption: Age Effects and Methodological Analyses," *Thyroid* 4, no. 1 (1994): 55–64.
3. P. R. Larsen and S. H. Ingbar, "The Thyroid Gland," in *Williams Textbook of Endocrinology*, 8th ed., J. F. Wilson and D. W. Foster eds. (Philadelphia, PA: W. B. Saunders, 1992): 357–487.
4. S. J. Mandel, G. A. Brent, and P. R. Larsen, "Levothyroxine Therapy in Patients with Thyroid Disease," *Annals of Internal Medicine* 119 (1993): 492–502.
5. E. Roti and L. E. Braverman, "Thyroid Hormone Therapy: When to Use It, When to Avoid It," *Drug Therapy* 24, no.4 (1994): 28–35.
6. G. Skinner et al., "Thyroxine Should Be Tried in Clinically Hypothyroid but Biochemically Euthyroid Patients," *British Medical Journal* 314 (1997): 1764–1765.

Step 4: Realize You May Still Be Low Thyroid Despite Normal Tests

1. R. D. Utiger, "Hypothyroidism," in *Endocrinology*, vol. 1, 2nd ed., ed I. J. DeGroot et al. (Philadelphia, PA: W. B. Saunders, 1989): 702–721.
2. W. Fraser et al., "Are Biochemical Tests of Thyroid Function of Any Value in Monitoring Patients Receiving Thyroxine Replacement?" *British Medical Journal*, (1986).
3. J. Hershman, "Getting the Most from Thyroid Tests," *Patient Care* (1989): 87–89.
4. R. Arem, *The Thyroid Solution* (New York: Ballantine Books, 1999): 224.
5. *Physicians' Desk Reference: A Medical Economics Publication* (Montvale, NJ: Medical Economics, 1999): 1123.
6. V. Nuzzo et al., "Bone Mineral Density in Premenopausal Women Receiving Levothyroxine Suppressive Therapy." *Gynecological Endocrinology* 12, no. 5 (1998): 333–337.

7. A. Lopez et al., "The Risk Factors and Bone Mineral Density in Women in Long-Term Levothyroxine Treatment," *Medical Clinics (Barcelona)* 112, no.3 (1999): 85–89.

Step 5: Discover Your Best Dose, Brand, or Mix of Medicines

1. R. Buneviciu et al., "Effects of Thyroxine As Compared with Thyroxine Plus Triiodothyronine in Patients with Hypothyroidism," *New England Journal of Medicine* 340 (1999): 424–429.
2. Ibid., 424–429.
3. R. Wilkinson, "Thyroid Function, Assessment, and Therapy," *University of Arizona Medical School Family Practice Review* (June 1998): 16.

Step 6: Reestablish Balance in Your Reproductive System

1. R. Arem, *The Thyroid Solution* (New York: Ballantine Books, 1999): 205.
2. A. J. Shelton et al., "Association Between Familial Autoimmune Diseases and Recurrent Spontaneous Abortions," *American Journal of Reproductive Immunology* 32, no. 2 (1994): 82–87.
3. I. Gerhard et al., "Thyroid and Ovarian Function in Infertile Women," *Human Reproduction* 6 (1991): 338–345.
4. R. Arem, *The Thyroid Solution* (New York: Ballantine Books, 1999): 200.
5. B. Barnes, *Hypothyroidism: The Unsuspected Illness* (New York: Harper and Row, 1976): 128–130.
6. L. Wood et al., *Your Thyroid: A Home Reference*, 3rd ed. (New York: Ballantine Books, 1995).

Step 7: Determine If Low Adrenal Should Also Be Treated

1. W. Jefferies, *Safe Uses of Cortisone* (Springfield: C. C. Thomas, 1981): 155–157.
2. A. Kasperlik-Zaluska, "High Prevalence of Thyroid Autoimmunity in Idiopathic Addison's Disease," *Autoimmunity* 18, no. 3 (1994): 213–216.
3. M. Laudat et al., "Salivary Cortisol Measurement: A Practical Approach to Assess Pituitary-Adrenal Function," *Journal of Clinical Endocrinology and Metabolism* 66, no. 2 (1988): 343.
4. J. Bolufer, "Salivary Corticosteroids in the Study of Adrenal Function," *Clinica Chimica Acta* 183 (1989): 217–226.
5. B. Kahn et al., "Salivary Cortisol: A Practical Method for Evaluation of Adrenal Function," *Biological Psychiatry* 23 (1988): 335–349.

Step 8: Boost Your Medication with Natural Therapies

1. P. Frame, "A Critical Review of Adult Health Maintenance," *Journal of Pharmacological Practice* 23 (1986): 29–39.

2. J. Kirshmann, *Nutrition Almanac*, 2nd ed. (New York: McGraw-Hill, 1984).

3. V. E. Kelley et al., "A Fish Oil Diet Rich in Eicosapentaenoic Acid Reduces Cycloxygenase Metabolites and Suppresses Lupus in MRL-1pr in Mice," *Journal of Immunology* 134 (1985): 1914–1919.

4. J. Ross, *The Diet Cure* (New York: Penguin Books, 2000).

5. J. Kirshmann, *Nutrition Almanac*, 2nd ed. (New York: McGraw-Hill, 1984).

6. S. Osborne, "Does Soy Have a Dark Side?" *Natural Health* (March 1999): 111–113, 157–158.

7. P. Galetti, and B. Goyet, "Effect of Fluorine in Thyroidal Iodine Metabolism in Hyperthyroidism," *Journal of Clinical Endocrinology* 18 (1958): 1102–1110.

8. J. Yiamouyiannis, *Flouride: The Aging Factor* (Delaware, OH: Health Action Press, 1993): 144.

9. M. Coplan and R. Masters, "Water Treatment with Silicofluorides and Lead Toxicity," *International Journal of Environmental Studies* 56 (1999): 435–449.

Step 9: Improve the Underlying Autoimmune Condition

1. Y. Tomer, "Infections and Autoimmune Endocrine Disease," *Baillieres Clin Endocrinol Metab* 9, no. 1 (1995): 47–70.

2. R. Arem, *The Thyroid Solution* (New York: Ballantine Books, 1999): 306.

3. T. Colburn, D. Dumanoski, and J. Myers, *Our Stolen Future* (New York: Dutton Publishing, 1996): 188.

4. M. Cone, "Human Immune Systems May Be Pollution Victims," *Los Angeles Times* (May 13, 1996): front page.

5. S. Krimsky, *Hormonal Chaos: The Scientific and Social Origins of the Environmental Endocrine Hypothesis* (Baltimore: Johns Hopkins University Press, 2000).

Further Reading

Thyroid-Related Books

Arem, R. *The Thyroid Solution*. New York: Ballantine Books, 1999.

Barnes, B. *Hypothyroidism: The Unsuspected Illness*. New York: Harper & Row, 1976.

Baskin, H. J. *How Your Thyroid Works*. Chicago: Adams Press, 1991.

Braverman, L., et al. *The Thyroid: A Fundamental Clinical Text*, 6th ed. Philadelphia: J. B. Lippincott, 1991.

Hamburger, J. *The Thyroid Gland*. Southfield, MI: J. Hamburger, 1991.

Jefferies, W. *Safe Uses of Cortisone*, 2nd ed. Springfield, IL: C. C. Thomas Publishers, 1996.

Langer, S. and J. Scheer. *Solved: The Riddle of Illness*. New Canaan, CT: Keats Publishing, 1995.

Ravicz, S. *Thriving with Your Autoimmune Disorder*. Oakland, CA: New Harbinger Publications, 2000.

Rosenthal, M. *The Thyroid Source Book*. Los Angeles, CA: Lowell House, 1996.

Rubenfeld, S. *Could It Be My Thyroid?* Houston, TX: S. Rubenfeld, 1996.

Shomon, M. *Living Well with Hypothyroidism*. New York: Avon Books, 2000.

Siegal, S. *Is Your Thyroid Making You Fat?* New York: Warner Books, 2000.

Teitelbaum, J. *From Fatigued to Fantastic*. Garden City Park, NY: Avery Publishing Group, 1996.

Volpe, R. *Autoimmunity in Endocrine Diseases*. Boca Raton: CRC Press, 1990.

Wilson, E. D. *Wilson's Syndrome*. Longwood, FL: Cornerstone Publishing, 1991.

Wood, L., et al. *Your Thyroid: A Home Reference*. New York: Ballantine Books, 1995.

Other Healing-Related Books

Bandura, A. *Self-Efficacy*. New York: W. H. Freeman, 1997.

Barash, M. and C. Hirshberg. *Remarkable Recovery*. New York: Putnam, 1995.

Carson, R. *Silent Spring*. New York: Houghton Mifflin, 1962.

Chopra, D. *Everyday Immortality*. New York: Crown Publishers, 1999.

Colburn, T, et al. *Our Stolen Future: Are We Threatening Our Fertility, Intelligence, & Survival?* New York: Dutton, 1996.

Diamond, J. *Male Menopause*. Naperville, IL: Sourcebooks, 1998.

Domar, A., and H. Dreher. *Healing Mind, Healthy Woman*. New York: Henry Holt, 1996.

Dossey, B. M., et al. *Holistic Nursing: A Handbook for Practice*, 2nd ed. Gaithersburg, MD: Aspen Publishers, 1995.

Dossey, L. *Healing Words*. San Francisco, CA: Harper SanFrancisco, 1993.

Earle, R., et al. *Your Vitality Quotient*. New York: Warner Books, 1989.

Ferguson, M. *The Aquarian Conspiracy*. Los Angeles, CA: J. P. Tarcher, 1980.

Fieve, R. *Mood Swing*. New York: Bantam Books, 1989.

Ford, G. *Listening to Your Hormones*. Rocklin, CA: Prima Publishing, 1997.

Garison, R. and E. Somer. *Nutrition Desk Reference*. New Canaan, CT: Keats, 1995.

Gerber, M. *Vibrational Medicine*. Santa Fe, NM: Bear & Co., 1988.

Hoffman, R. *Tired All the Time: How to Regain Your Lost Energy*. New York: Pocket Books, 1993.

Hover-Kramer, D. and K. Shames. *Energetic Approaches to Emotional Healing*. Albany, NY: Delmar Publishers, 1997.

Keegan, L. and G. Keegan. *Healing Waters: The Miraculous Health Benefits of Earth's Most Essential Resource.* New York: Berkley Books, 1998.

Krimsky, S. *Hormonal Chaos: The Scientific and Social Origins of the Environmental Endocrine Hypothesis.* Baltimore, MD: Johns Hopkins Press, 2000.

Kubler-Ross, E. *On Death and Dying.* New York: Simon & Schuster, 1997.

Laskow, L. *Healing with Love.* New York: HarperCollins, 1992.

Lee, J. *What Your Doctor May Not Tell You About Menopause.* New York: Warner Books, 1996.

Love, S. *Dr. Susan Love's Hormone Book.* New York: Random House, 1997.

Mathews-Larson, J. *Seven Weeks to Sobriety.* New York: Ballantine, 1992.

Murray, M. *Premenstrual Syndrome.* Rocklin, CA: Prima, 1997.

Nightingale, F. *Notes on Nursing.* London: Harrison & Sons, 1860.

Northrup, C. *Women's Bodies, Women's Wisdom.* New York: Bantam, 1998.

Page, L. *Healthy Healing: A Guide to Self-Healing for Everyone,* 10th ed. Healthy Healing Publishers, 1997.

Pert, C. *Molecules of Emotion.* New York: Scribner, 1997.

Randolph, T. *An Alternative Approach to Allergies.* New York: HarperCollins, 1989.

Rapp, D. *Is This Your Child?* New York: William Morrow, 1991.

Ross, J. *The Diet Cure: An 8-Step Program to Rebalance Your Body Chemistry.* New York: Viking, 1999.

Rossman, M. *Healing Yourself: A Step by Step Program for Better Health Through Imagery.* New York: Walker, 1987.

Schaef, A. W. *Beyond Therapy, Beyond Science: A New Model for Healing the Whole Person.* San Francisco, CA: HarperSanFrancisco, 1992.

Shames, K. *Creative Imagery in Nursing.* Albany, NY: Delmar Publishers, 1996.

Selye, H. *The Stress of Life.* New York: McGraw Hill, 1956.

Shames, K. *The Nightingale Conspiracy.* Montclair, NJ: Enlightenment Press, 1993.

Shames, R. and K. Shames. *The Gift of Health.* New York: Bantam Books, 1982.

Shames, R. and C. Sterin. *Healing with Mind Power.* Emmaus, PA: Rodale Press, 1978.

Somer, E. *Food & Mood.* New York: Henry Holt, 1995.

Steingraber, S. *Living Downstream: A Scientist's Personal Investigation of Cancer and the Environment.* New York: Random House, 1998.

Vliet, E. L. *Screaming to Be Heard: Hormonal Connections Women Suspect and Doctors Ignore.* New York: M. Evan, 1995.

Weil, A. *8 Weeks to Optimal Health.* Old Tappan, NJ: MacMillan Library References, 1997.

Wright, J. *Natural Hormone Replacement for Women Over 45*. Seattle, WA: Smart
     Publications, 1997.

Yiamouyiannis, J. *Fluoride: The Aging Factor*. Delaware, OH: Health Action
     Press, 1993.

Thyroid-Related Articles

Bailes, B. K. "Hypothyroidism in elderly patients." *AORN Journal* 69(5):
     1026–30 (1999).

Borges, M. F., et al. "Calcitonin deficiency: early stages of chronic autoimmune
     thyroiditis." *Clinical Endocrinology* (Oxf) 49(1):69–75 (1998).

Caffarra, P., et al. "Ataxia and hypothyroidism." *Italian Journal of Neurological
     Sciences* 7(6):625 (1986).

Coleman, R. and R. J. Hay. "Chronic mucocutaneous candidiasis associated
     with hypothyroidism: a distinct syndrome?" *British Journal of Dermatology*
     136(1):24–9 (1997).

Coser, P. et al. "Thrombotic thrombocytopenic purpura in hypothyroidism: an
     accidental association?" *Haematologica* 67(4):625–9 (1982).

Frankton S. et al. "Pituitary-thyroid feedback hypersensitivity as a novel cause of
     hypothyroidism in children." *The Lancet* 356: 1238–40 (2000).

Ghayad, E. et al. "Scleroderma with anomalies of the thyroid function. 7 Cases."
     Annals Medicine Internel (Paris) 148(4):307–10 (1997).

Gold, M. S., A. L. Pottash, and I. Extein. "Hypothyroidism and depression. Evi-
     dence from complete thyroid function evaluation." *JAMA* 245(19):1919–22
     (1981).

Green, S. T. and J. P. Ng. "Hypothyroidism and anaemia." *Biomedical Pharma-
     cotherapy* 40(9):326–31(1986).

Guerin, V. et al. "Dysthyroidism and Parkinson's disease." *Annals of Endocrinol-
     ogy* 51(1): 43–5 (1990).

Hak, E. et al. "Subclinical hypothyroidism is an independent risk factor for ath-
     erosclerosis and myocardial infarction in elderly women: The Rotterdam
     Study." *Annals of Internal Medicine* 132 (4): 691–97 (2000).

Hess, R. S. and C. R. Ward. "Diabetes mellitus, hyperadrenocorticism, and
     hypothyroidism in a dog." *Journal of the American Animal Hospital Association*
     34(3):204–7 (1998).

Johannessen, A. C. et al. "Thyroid function in patients with Parkinson's disease."
     Acta Neurol Scand 75(5): 364–5 (1987).

Keenan, G. F. et al. "Rheumatic symptoms associated with hypothyroidism in children." *Journal of Pediatrics* 123(4):586–8 (1993).

Krupsky, M. et al. "Musculoskeletal symptoms as a presenting sign of long-standing hypothyroidism." *Israel Journal of Medical Science* 23(11):1110–3 (1987).

Kunisada, K. et al. "Case of hypothyroidism and hypoparathyroidism discovered by fainting spells." *Nippon Naika Gakkai Zasshi* 87(11): 2314–5 (1998).

Lanigan, S. W. et al. "Association between urticaria and hypothyroidism." *Lancet* 1(8392):1476 (1994).

Leung, A. S. et al. "Perinatal outcome in hypothyroid pregnancies." *Obstetrics & Gynecology* 81(3):349–53 (1993).

Lopez, A. et al. "Sleep apnea, hypothyroidism and pulmonary edema." *Chest.* 97(3):763–4 (1990).

McLean, R. M. and D. N. Podell. "Bone and joint manifestations of hypothyroidism." *Seminars Arthritis Rheumatology* 24(4):282–90 (1995).

Mullin, G. E. and J. S. Eastern. "Cutaneous signs of thyroid disease." *American Family Physician* 34(4):93–8 (1986).

Neeck G., and W. Riedel. "Neuropathy, myopathy and destructive arthropathy in primary hypothyroidism." *Journal of Rheumatology* 17(12)1697–700 (1990).

Pauszek, M. E. "Hypertension as the presenting problem in primary hypothyroidism." *Indiana Medical Journal* 82(1):28–9 (1989).

Rowe, M. S. et al. "Hypothyroidism with coexistent asthma: problems in management." *Southern Medical Journal* 77(3):401–2 (1984).

Rumbyrt, J. S. et al. "Resolution of chronic urticaria in patients with thyroid autoimmunity." *Journal of Allergy & Clinical Immunology* 96(6 Pt 1):901–5 (1995).

Skinner, G. R. B. et al. "Thyroxine should be tried in clinically hypothyroid but biochemically Euthyroid patients." *British Medical Journal* 314: 1764 (1997).

Sridhar, G. R. and G. Nagamani. "Hypothyroidism presenting with polycystic ovary syndrome." *Journal of the Association of Physicians in India* 41(2):88–90 (1993).

Wiesli, P. et al. "Headache and bilateral visual loss in a young hypothyroid Indian man." *Journal of Endocrinological Investigation* 22(2):141–3 (1999).

Yamada, T. "Manic-depressive symptom associated with endocrine and metabolic disorders." *Nippon Rinsho* 52(5):1311–17 (1994).

Yokoe, T. et al. "Relationship between thyroid-pituitary function and response to therapy in patients with recurrent breast cancer." *Anticancer Research* 16(4A):2069–72 (1996).

Index